CHANGING HEALTH BEHAVIOUR

CHANGING HEALTH BEHAVIOUR
INTERVENTION AND RESEARCH
WITH SOCIAL COGNITION MODELS

Edited by
Derek Rutter and Lyn Quine

Open University Press
Buckingham · Philadelphia

Open University Press
Celtic Court
22 Ballmoor
Buckingham
MK18 1XW

email: enquiries@openup.co.uk
world wide web: www.openup.co.uk

and
325 Chestnut Street
Philadelphia, PA 19106, USA

First Published 2002

A catalogue record of this book is available from the British Library

ISBN   0 335 20432 5 (pb)   0 335 20433 3 (hb)

Library of Congress Cataloging-in-Publication Data
Changing health behaviour: intervention and research with social cognition models/edited by Derek Rutter and Lyn Quine.
    p. cm.
  Includes bibliographical references and index.
  ISBN 0-335-20433-3 – ISBN 0-335-20432-5 (pbk.)
    1. Health behavior.   2. Health attitudes.   3. Social perception.
  4. Behavior modification.   I. Rutter, D.R. (Derek R.)   II. Quine, Lyn.

RA776.9 .C437 2002
613–dc21
                                  2001036115

Typeset by Graphicraft Limited, Hong Kong
Printed in Great Britain by Biddles Limited, Guildford and King's Lynn

CONTENTS

LIST OF CONTRIBUTORS

Professor Charles Abraham is Professor of Psychology at the Centre for Research in Health and Medicine (CRHaM), University of Sussex.

Dr Christopher Armitage is Lecturer in Social and Health Psychology at the Department of Psychology, University of Sheffield.

Dr Laurence Arnold recently completed his PhD at the Department of Psychology, University of Kent at Canterbury.

Dr Mark Conner is Reader in Applied Social Psychology at the School of Psychology, University of Leeds.

Dr Daphne Evans recently completed her PhD at the Department of Psychology, University of Wales, Swansea.

Susie Frost is a clinical research worker at the Eating Disorders Research Unit, Institute of Psychiatry, King's College London.

Dr Lynn B. Myers is Lecturer in Health Psychology at the Department of Psychiatry and Behavioural Sciences, University College London.

Dr Paul Norman is Senior Lecturer in Psychology at the Department of Psychology, University of Sheffield.

Professor Sheina Orbell is Professor of Psychology at the Department of Psychology, University of Essex.

Dr Dianne Parker is Senior Lecturer in Social Psychology at the Department of Psychology, University of Manchester.

Dr Lyn Quine is Reader in Health Psychology at the Department of Psychology, University of Kent at Canterbury.

Professor Derek Rutter is Professor of Health Psychology at the Department of Psychology, University of Kent at Canterbury.

Dr Peter M. Sandman, formerly Director of the Environmental Communication Research Program at Rutgers University, now runs a risk communication consultancy based in Princeton, New Jersey, USA.

Professor Sue Scott is Professor of Sociology at the Department of Sociology and Social Policy at the University of Durham.

Dr Paschal Sheeran is Reader in Psychology at the Department of Psychology, University of Sheffield.

Professor Stephen Sutton is Professor of Behavioural Science at the Institute of Public Health, University of Cambridge.

Professor Jane Wardle is Professor of Clinical Psychology at the Department of Epidemiology and Public Health, University College London, and Director of the Imperial Cancer Research Fund's Health Behaviour Unit.

Dr Neil D. Weinstein is Professor of Human Ecology at the Department of Human Ecology, Rutgers University, New Brunswick, New Jersey.

Dr Daniel Wight is a senior researcher at the Medical Research Council's Social and Public Health Sciences Unit, University of Glasgow.

Sara Williamson is a research psychologist at the Imperial Cancer Research Fund's Health Behaviour Unit in the Department of Epidemiology and Public Health, University College London.

ACKNOWLEDGEMENT

We are delighted once again to have the opportunity to thank our secretary, Jo Oven. Jo has worked with us for many years and has been copy editor-in-chief for this and all our other publications since she joined us. Somehow, along the way, she has also found time to complete her PhD on the concept of human nature in vernacular writers of the French Renaissance. Congratulations and thank you, Dr Oven.

LIST OF ABBREVIATIONS

ALA	American Lung Association
BSE	breast self-examination
CDC	Centers for Disease Control
DAQ	Driver Attitude Questionnaire
DETR	Department of the Environment, Transport and the Regions
ELM	Elaboration Likelihood Model
FOBT	faecal occult blood testing
FS	flexible sigmoidoscopy
GP	general practitioner
HBM	Health Belief Model
HIV	human immunodeficiency virus
MAFF	Ministry of Agriculture, Fisheries and Food
NRT	Nicotine Replacement Therapy
PACTS	Parliamentary Advisory Council for Traffic Safety
PAPM	Precaution Adoption Process Model
PBC	perceived behavioural control
PCB	perceived control over behaviour
RCOG	Royal College of Obstetricians and Gynaecologists
RCT	randomised controlled trial
STD	sexually transmitted disease
STI	sexually transmitted infection
TPB	Theory of Planned Behaviour
TRA	Theory of Reasoned Action
TSE	testicular self-examination
TTM	Transtheoretical Model

<table>
<tr><td>1</td><td>DEREK RUTTER AND
LYN QUINE</td></tr>
</table>

SOCIAL COGNITION MODELS AND CHANGING HEALTH BEHAVIOURS

1 Social cognition models

For many years, social psychological models have been at the forefront of research into predicting and explaining health behaviours. The most frequently used have been social cognition models. Until recently, however, there were few attempts to go beyond prediction and understanding to *intervention* – the systematic attempt to change people's health behaviours – but since the mid-1990s the position has changed, and there are now a number of very good, theory-driven, interventions in progress. As yet, so far as we know, there has been no attempt to bring the research together, and it is for that reason that we have produced this edited book. We have tried to include a representative cross-section of research, in that each chapter takes a particular health behaviour (sometimes more than one) and uses a particular theoretical model or framework to design and carry out the intervention. We hope that the book will appeal to academics, health professionals, and advanced students in psychology and health-related disciplines.

The starting point for the book is social cognition theory. Definitions of social cognition may vary, but the central tenet is that people's social behaviour is best understood by examining their beliefs about their behaviour in a social context, and their social perceptions and representations. Recognition of the term probably stems from the reconceptualization of social psychology that took place in the late 1960s and early 1970s. Social psychologists had struggled to demonstrate the links between attitudes and behaviour that tradition had accepted must exist, and they turned to new concepts and models for solutions, among them the young Theory of Reasoned Action (Fishbein and Ajzen 1975). 'Social cognition' quickly became a distinctive and accepted term, and research developed apace to make the area one of the fastest growing in the discipline. By the mid-1990s, the role of social cognition models in helping to understand and predict *health* behaviours was well established in the literature, and the principal models and health-related research that each had inspired were brought together for the first time in *Predicting Health Behaviour*, edited by Mark Conner and Paul Norman, which was published by Open University Press in 1996.

The purpose of Conner and Norman (1996) was to provide an integrated and critical review of the main social cognition models and the research in health behaviour that had been published within each of the frameworks. The chapters were contributed by specialists and covered five widely used approaches: the Health Belief Model, Health Locus of Control, Protection Motivation Theory, the Theory of Planned Behaviour and Self-Efficacy. Each chapter ended with speculations about future directions. Since then, a number of developments have taken place in the literature, and they are discussed in this chapter and elsewhere in the book. First, there have been new critical reviews, some organized by model and some by behaviour. Second, there have been meta-analyses, which allow results from all the available studies that reach the author's methodological criteria to be combined statistically. Third, several writers have explored ways of modifying the existing models, or adding variables to them, in an effort to strengthen and clarify the prediction and understanding of health behaviours. And, fourth, the first interventions designed to modify health behaviours through the application of social cognition models have been designed and preliminary findings have begun to appear.

It is the purpose of this book to report some of the most important interventions that have been recently completed or are in progress. We have chosen to organize the material by behaviour, but each empirical chapter is intended to stand alone. Like Conner and Norman, we have asked contributors to follow a common format. Each chapter begins with a statement of the 'epidemiological facts' about the health problem it addresses, and describes the links between the behaviour in question and outcome. It then outlines the theoretical stance the chapter takes, generally by describing the particular form of the model it employs. The authors then report their intervention or interventions, and the chapter ends with a discussion of the implications of the findings for theory, policy and practice. The one exception to the common format is the concluding chapter, by Stephen Sutton – a final reflection on the problems that authors face and the assumptions they make in using social cognition models to develop health behaviour interventions.

2 The empirical chapters

The body of the book consists of nine empirical chapters, each concerned with a particular behaviour or set of behaviours. Chapters 2 to 4 examine risk-related behaviours (safer sex; smoking; exposure to radon gas); Chapters 5 to 7 turn to health-enhancing behaviours and screening (reducing fat intake; uptake of vitamin C; breast self-examination; participation in cervical and colorectal cancer screening); and Chapters 8 to 10 explore road safety (speeding by drivers; pedestrian behaviour; cycle helmet use). In this section of the introductory chapter, we outline the aims and objectives of the studies, and in the following section we introduce the models on which the interventions are based.

Chapter 2 is by Charles Abraham, Daniel Wight and Sue Scott. It describes a large-scale, schools-based intervention designed to encourage safer-sex behaviours. The median age for first sexual encounters continues to fall, and substantial numbers of young people are putting themselves at risk of sexually transmitted infections. The case for interventions to improve sex education and encourage safer-sex behaviours is strong and clear, but there has been little investment in setting up and testing theory-driven programmes. The SHARE project (Sexual Health and Relationships: Safe Happy and Responsible), the subject of the chapter, is a notable exception. It is currently being tested and developed in secondary schools in eastern Scotland, and it is based in the classroom. It includes a five-day training course for the teachers who deliver it, together with a teachers' resource pack of twenty sessions, and it takes place over two school years. Its theoretical base is symbolic interactionism and script theory – not encountered elsewhere in the book – and among the themes of the intervention are discussion, negotiation, sexual identity and agency. Outcome data are not yet available – the effects of the programme on young people's behaviour – but the chapter reports preliminary findings from first experiences of delivering the programme, and discusses implications for testing and developing it further.

Chapter 3 is by Lynn B. Myers and Susie Frost, and reports an intervention designed to encourage smokers to quit. Smoking is one of the world's most pressing health problems, and it is estimated that, across the globe, 450 million people alive today will die of smoking-related illnesses over the next 50 years. The benefits to the individual of quitting, however late, are considerable – the risk of lung cancer falls by 50 per cent over 10 years, for example – yet the success rates of interventions are seldom high. Two strategies have predominated: motivational (to strengthen smokers' attempts to give up) and treatment (to support abstinence by helping to overcome the effects of nicotine withdrawal, through nicotine patches and the like). The authors' intervention is motivational, and seeks to modify what smokers believe about the risks of contracting smoking-related diseases by attacking their 'unrealistic optimism' and helping them to see the risks as they really are. The work is based on asking participants to imagine scenarios in which they develop the disease and have to think about the consequences for their lives – personal, social and work alike. The results so far have differed markedly according to how optimistically biased respondents were before the intervention started. The dependent measure was how much people's beliefs changed, and the findings showed an unexpected pattern: those who were optimistically biased at the outset became less optimistic, but those who were not became *more* optimistic. The implication is that interventions must be carefully tailored to people's initial positions.

Chapter 4 is by Neil D. Weinstein and Peter M. Sandman, and takes the argument about individual tailoring one step further. It reports a field experiment designed to encourage people to test their homes for radon gas. The basis of the intervention is Weinstein's own Precaution Adoption Process Model (PAPM), and the chapter is an instructive example of the cyclical way in which theory leads to experimental intervention, which leads back in turn to modifications to theory. Radon is a radioactive gas produced by the decaying uranium found naturally in the soil. In the USA, it is the leading cause of lung cancer after smoking. The PAPM, a stage theory, has been used to analyse a variety of health behaviours, and argues that people will be persuaded to change only if the message is matched to the stage they have reached in their thinking: unaware of the issue, unengaged, deciding about acting, decided not to act, decided to act, acting, and maintenance. The chapter focuses on two transitions: unengaged to deciding, and deciding to acting (in this case ordering a radon testing kit). The intervention was based on videos, and strong support for the model and the approach to interventions was found: there was good evidence for distinct stages; and stage-matched attacks, though expensive to produce, succeeded where others did not.

Chapter 5 is by Christopher J. Armitage and Mark Conner. It is the first of the chapters on health-enhancing behaviours, and it reports an intervention to encourage people to reduce their intake of fat. Excessive fat is known to be associated with many disorders, including heart disease and cancer, and guidelines have been produced in several countries. In the UK, for example, the recommendation is that no more than 35 per cent of food energy should come from fat, and no more than 11 per cent from saturated fat, but the average has remained above these figures for 20 years or more and shows little sign of falling. The authors' intervention was based on their newly extended version of Ajzen's Theory of Planned Behaviour (TPB), and used a randomized control design. Fat intake was measured at Time 1; three months later participants underwent one of three interventions (TPB, self-efficacy, or plain information), and five months later still their fat intake was measured again. All three interventions used leaflets. Both the TPB and self-efficacy conditions had a small effect on total fat intake across the whole group, but all three led to a reduction among people whose normal intake was high. Thus, against prediction, all conditions produced measurable effects on behaviour; but the two theory-driven conditions were more successful than the information-only control.

Chapter 6 is by Sara Williamson and Jane Wardle, and reports an intervention to increase uptake of a new bowel cancer screening test, flexible sigmoidoscopy. Bowel cancer is one of the most common causes of cancer death in the UK and most of Europe, and in the USA. Survival rates are low but, if the disease is detected early and the pre-cancerous polyps are removed, the chance of survival is much enhanced. Flexible sigmoidoscopy (FS) allows both detection and removal, and is the current approach of choice, but uptake is low. The authors' purpose was to try to increase uptake by means of an intervention based on the Health Belief Model. The study was conducted as part of a UK national trial of FS, and used a booklet designed to reduce perceptions of barriers and increase positive beliefs among people who had declared themselves 'probably interested' in attending if offered the chance. The booklet acknowledged potential barriers, suggested possible coping strategies, allowed participants to rehearse the benefits of screening, and directed their attention to the positive emotional impact of screening. It also provided normative information and modelled ways of seeking social support. Participants were assigned at random to 'booklet' and 'no booklet' conditions, and it was found that screening intention was influenced markedly – 42.5 per cent said they were 'very likely' to attend after the intervention, against 29.4 per cent in the control condition. Whether intention has translated into action will be known shortly.

Chapter 7 is by Sheina Orbell and Paschal Sheeran. It takes a different approach from other chapters in that it reports three interventions, but all are based on the one concept, implementation intentions. The health issues addressed are practising breast self-examination (BSE), using vitamin C supplements, and attending for cervical screening. Social cognition models are generally about the *motivational* phase of planning behaviour, the processes up to intention, and stop short of trying to bridge the gap to behaviour, the post-decisional *volitional* phase. What Orbell and Sheeran do is try to increase the probability that the behaviour will occur by intervening to make people plan when and where they will execute the behaviour itself – the process of forming implementation intentions. Their technique is simple – ask participants to write down their plan and commit themselves to it – and the findings were striking. In the BSE study, 100 per cent of intenders who underwent the intervention subsequently examined themselves, against 53 per cent of intenders in the control condition; in the cervical screening study, attendance rates were 92 per cent and 69 per cent; and in the vitamin C study, significantly fewer experimental participants than controls missed pills. Interventions using implementation intentions are both cheap and easy to conduct, and these first applications to health behaviours indicate that they produce strong and reliable results.

Chapter 8 is by Dianne Parker and is the first of the final group of three, on road safety. One of the most important contributors to road traffic accidents and to serious injuries is driving too fast. Speeding has been estimated to be second only to drink-driving as a cause and is known to be directly associated with accident death rates. Many governments impose speed limits, of course, but failure to respect them is widespread, is seldom punished severely, and is socially acceptable to many people. The intervention reported in this chapter followed a long programme of research to identify the beliefs and values that distinguish drivers who report committing violations on the road, including speeding, from those who do not. It was based on the TPB, and its purpose was to persuade drivers to slow down. Four short videos were made, each designed to change beliefs, attitudes and intentions associated with driving at 40 m.p.h. in a 30 m.p.h. area. One concentrated on behavioural beliefs, another normative beliefs, another perceived behavioural control, and another anticipated regret. All showed the same central character driving too fast along a quiet residential road and being assailed by triggers – in the normative condition, for example, members of his family and salient others disapproving of his speeding. The main outcome measure was responses to the Driver Attitude Questionnaire, a standardized index of general attitude to driving violations, and the strongest response was found for anticipated regret. This is a variable that has recently been used by the author and others to extend the TPB, and the chapter thus provides a good example of something we pointed out earlier – the way in which experimental interventions can make not only a *practical* contribution but a *theoretical* one too, testing theory and exploring ways of extending and improving it.

Chapter 9 is by Daphne Evans and Paul Norman, and turns to adolescent pedestrians. One child in fifteen is injured on the roads of Britain before the age of 16, and children aged 10 to 15 have the highest road casualty rate of the whole population. The intervention was based again on the TPB, but this time made use of theatre and drama. In the drama condition, 11–12-year-olds worked with their teacher to produce a 15-minute play about crossing the road safely, using information provided by the authors and their own observations of how they and their peers behaved as pedestrians. In the theatre condition, children of the same age watched the play as the drama class performed it. Both groups completed TPB questionnaires before and after the intervention, including items on additional variables that the authors used to supplement the model – moral norm, anticipated regret and self-identity. The theatre intervention produced changes in both behavioural and normative beliefs, while the drama condition influenced both perceived behavioural control and intention. The implications are that school-based interventions have considerable potential, and that active engagement is the key.

Chapter 10 is by Lyn Quine, Derek Rutter and Laurence Arnold, and completes the empirical chapters with an examination of cycle helmet use among children riding to and from school. Deaths and injuries among school-age cyclists between 8 and 19 account for almost 40 per cent of all injuries to cyclists in Britain – and are probably under-reported. Accidents are most likely to occur during school journeys on weekdays, and the injuries are often to the head and brain. Helmets are known to reduce the risk of head, face and brain injury by up to 90 per cent, yet few school-age cyclists wear them. The chapter reports an intervention based once more on the Theory of Planned Behaviour, but using techniques from the Elaboration Likelihood Model of Persuasion to encourage systematic thinking about the message. The purpose of the intervention was to persuade non-wearers to become wearers. The participants were adolescents who rode to school regularly but did not wear a helmet. Participants were randomly assigned to intervention or control conditions. Initial beliefs were measured just before the intervention at Time 1. In the intervention condition, participants carried out two paper and pencil tasks, both of them designed to encourage recall and elaboration of salient beliefs about wearing a helmet: completing word and picture flow charts; and thought listing. In the control condition, participants were given similar materials and tasks, but this time concerned with a hypothetical cycling proficiency and maintenance course. The immediate effects of the intervention on attitude, subjective norm, control beliefs and intention were measured after the intervention at Time 2. Five months later, at Time 3, the long-term effects of the intervention on beliefs, intentions and behaviours were measured. It was found that 25 per cent of the intervention group were now wearing their helmets against none of the control group. There was good evidence that the difference was associated with belief change. While the intervention was time-consuming to conduct, incorporating it routinely into cycling proficiency training would be both easy and cost-effective.

3 The theoretical models

In this section of the chapter, we turn to the models or theoretical approaches on which the empirical chapters are based. A number of the authors have used extended or variant forms of the models, and they explain their choices and amendments in their own chapters. Our purpose in this chapter is to outline the original forms of the models and to indicate some of the ways in which they have been used in the literature. There are five approaches to discuss: risk perception and optimistic bias; the Health Belief Model; the Theory of Planned Behaviour; implementation intentions; and stage models.

3.1 Risk perception and optimistic bias

The literature on risk perception and optimistic bias owes most, perhaps, to Neil Weinstein. Weinstein (1980) drew attention to what he called the 'popular belief' that people tend to think they are invulnerable. We generally expect misfortunes to happen to others, he argued, not ourselves, and most members of a group will say they are less likely than the average to suffer the bad things in life and more likely than the average to experience the good things. The bias holds for a wide range of health and other outcomes, from the trivial (being ill in bed for a day or two, or having a tooth extracted) to the life threatening (having a heart attack, or being involved in a road accident). The name he coined for the bias was 'unrealistic optimism'.

Since Weinstein's first papers (Weinstein 1980, 1982, 1983, 1984, 1987), a considerable literature on unrealistic optimism has developed, and many useful reviews have been published (see for example Perloff and Fetzer 1986; Hoorens 1994; Schwarzer 1994; Van der Pligt 1994; Taylor and Armor 1996; Weinstein and Klein 1996; Van der Pligt 1998). Once descriptive research had made clear the extent of the bias, attention turned to a variety of theoretical issues, of which two in particular have recurred in the literature. The first is where the bias comes from, its origins in people's motives and cognitions, and the ways in which it may be mediated by experience. For Weinstein, the most likely *motivational* candidates were defensiveness and wishful thinking, but overall he gave more weight to *cognitive* factors. Thus, the more probable I believe an event to be, he argued, the more likely I am to believe that its probability for me is greater than average; the more I believe I can control a negative event, the more I will perceive my own probability as less than average; and if I have personal experience of the negative event, I am more likely to perceive its future probability for me as greater than average. Controllability (Van der Velde *et al.* 1992; McKenna 1993; Harris and Middleton 1994; Harris 1996; Hoorens 1996; Myers and Reynolds 2000), the debiasing effects of experience (Dolinski *et al.* 1987; Van der Pligt 1991; Van der Velde and Van der Pligt 1991; Burger and Palmer 1992; McKenna and Albery 2001) and experimental interventions to produce debiasing (Kreuter and Strecher 1995; Weinstein and Klein 1995; Stapel and Velthuijsen 1996; McKenna and Myers 1997) have all generated extensive literatures.

The second issue has been whether unrealistic optimism predicts behaviour. Weinstein (1989) argued that it probably does, or at least that it ought to, but that the literature has been bedevilled by conceptual and methodological problems. Chief among them is that most of the analyses have been cross-sectional or retrospective, so that respondents report their risk perceptions on the same occasion as their concurrent or even past behaviour (see, for example, Svenson *et al.* 1985; Dolinski *et al.* 1987; Weinstein *et al.* 1990; Weinstein and Nicolich 1993; Hoorens 1994; Gerrard *et al.* 1996).

As Van der Pligt (1994) argued, *prospective* studies are essential if causal ordering is to be disentangled, but relatively few have been reported and the results have been inconsistent (see the review by Hoorens 1994). Moreover, Otten and Van der Pligt (1992) have suggested that unrealistic optimism is in any case a much less powerful predictor than prior behaviour. There are two reasons, they argue: first, prior behaviour affects subsequent behaviour directly (Bentler and Speckart 1979); and second, perceptions of risk are themselves a product of prior behaviour, and their role is at most to *mediate* its effects. Thus, prior behaviour will absorb most of the variance, and any apparent effect of risk perception is likely to be less a 'pure' effect of perceived risk than an indirect effect of prior behaviour. Once again, if an *experimental* approach is not feasible, the most useful alternative is a prospective longitudinal design.

3.2 The Health Belief Model

The Health Belief Model (HBM: Rosenstock 1966, 1974a, 1974b) proposes that people will be motivated to carry out preventive health behaviours in response to a perceived threat to their health (see Figure 1.1). Two classes of variables are important: '(1) the psychological state of readiness to take specific action, and (2) the extent to which a particular course of action is believed to be beneficial in reducing the threat' (Rosenstock 1966: 98). Both variables, Rosenstock argued, are two-dimensional. The individual's

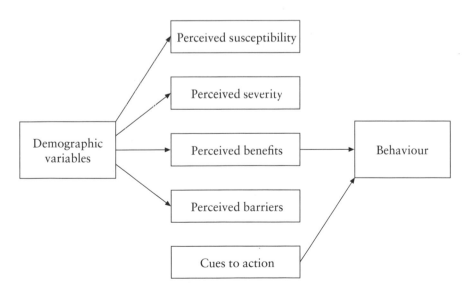

Figure 1.1 The Health Belief Model

state of readiness to act is determined by perceptions of personal susceptibility or *vulnerability* to a particular health threat, *and* perceptions of the
severity with which that threat might affect their life. The extent to which a
course of action is believed to be beneficial is the result of beliefs about the
benefits to be gained by a particular action weighed against the costs of or
barriers to action. Rosenstock (1966: 101) believed that the level of readiness provided the energy or force to act and the perceptions of benefits less
barriers provided a preferred path of action. However, the combination of
these could reach considerable levels of intensity without resulting in overt
action unless some instigating event occurred to set the process in motion
or trigger action in an individual psychologically ready to act (Rosenstock
1966: 102). Thus, in addition to the variables already described, a factor
that serves as a cue or a trigger to appropriate action is necessary – such
as having an accident oneself (in the case of road safety, for example), or
recent media attention to the issue. This Rosenstock named the 'cue to
action'. Some years later, Rosenstock and his colleagues also suggested that
behavioural intention might be a mediating variable between the components of the HBM and behaviour (Becker *et al.* 1977). Other researchers have
taken up this suggestion (King 1982; Calnan 1984; Norman and Fitter 1989;
Quine *et al.* 1998).

Despite its intuitive appeal, the HBM has conceptual difficulties. Rosenstock did not specify how different beliefs influence one another, or how
the explanatory variables combine to influence behaviour. As a result, different studies have used different combinations of variables, and researchers
have treated variables differently in the analysis. Some, for example, have
used additive models in which the combined weight of the variables is
used to predict outcome, while others have combined variables – by adding
vulnerability and severity (Wyper 1990; Witte *et al.* 1993), multiplying them
(Haefner and Kirscht 1970; Hill *et al.* 1985; Conner and Norman 1994) or
subtracting barriers from benefits (Oliver and Berger 1979; Rutledge 1987;
Wyper 1990). A close inspection of Rosenstock's discussion of the model,
however, seems to indicate that the dimensions are to be treated as separate influences on health behaviour and that an additive combination is consistent with the underlying theoretical principles (see Weinstein 1988 for
a discussion).

A second problem is that Rosenstock offered no operational definitions
of the variables and therefore researchers use different methods (Champion
1984). Perceived vulnerability is used to measure either personal vulnerability to a specific health threat or a general vulnerability to disease relative
to other people. Barriers, which Rosenstock viewed as primarily psychological, are often used to assess structural impediments instead (Hill *et al.*
1985; Melnyk 1988; Simon *et al.* 1993). Several revisions to the model
have therefore been suggested (Becker *et al.* 1972; Becker and Maiman
1975; Becker *et al.* 1977). Becker (1974) has argued that the value placed

upon their health by some individuals may predispose them to respond to the cues to action. Some researchers have suggested that health locus of control beliefs should be included (Wallston and Wallston 1981; Lau *et al.* 1986; Arnold and Quine 1994). Others have produced new conceptual frameworks using some of the HBM's constructs: see Schwarzer (1992), Schwarzer and Fuchs (1996), Schwarzer (1999) (the Health Action Process Approach); Rogers (1975, 1985), Prentice-Dunn and Rogers (1986), Boer and Seydel (1996) (Protection Motivation Theory).

Despite these theoretical and conceptual problems, the HBM has received sustained empirical support and is still widely used to predict health behaviours. Since the early 1990s, for example, it has been applied to mammography and cervical screening (Aiken *et al.* 1994; Fischera and Frank 1994; Champion and Miller 1996; Orbell *et al.* 1996; Brenes and Skinner 1999); breast self-examination (Champion 1990; Friedman *et al.* 1994; Savage and Clarke 1996; Millar 1997); adherence to medication (Budd *et al.* 1996; Hughes *et al.* 1997; Nageotte *et al.* 1997) (antipsychotic medication), (Brown and Segal 1996) (antihypertensive medication), (Bond *et al.* 1992) (insulin), (Abraham *et al.* 1999) (malaria medication); exercise behaviour (Corwyn and Benda 1999); safe-sex behaviours (Petosa and Jackson 1991; Abraham *et al.* 1992; Walter *et al.* 1993; Lux and Petosa 1994; Steers *et al.* 1996; Bakker *et al.* 1997); attendance at health checks (Norman and Conner 1993); delay in seeking medical care (Leenaars *et al.* 1993) (sexually transmitted infections: STIs), (Dracup *et al.* 1995) (heart attack); and many other health behaviours. Two reviews using rather different methods have examined the utility of the Health Belief Model constructs (see Janz and Becker 1984; Harrison *et al.* 1992). These are evaluated in Sheeran and Abraham (1996), who concluded that though the HBM constructs are frequently significant predictors of behaviour, their effects are usually small.

3.3 The Theory of Planned Behaviour

The TPB is an expectancy-value model that was expanded from the Theory of Reasoned Action (TRA: Fishbein and Ajzen 1975; Ajzen and Fishbein 1980) (see Figure 1.2). It provides a theoretical account of the way in which attitude, subjective norm and behavioural intentions combine to predict behaviour. According to the TRA, the best predictor of behaviour is the person's intention to perform the behaviour (for example 'I intend to do X'). Intention summarizes the individual's motivation to behave in a particular way and indicates how hard the person is willing to try and how much time and effort they are prepared to expend in order to perform the behaviour (Ajzen 1991: 199). In turn, intention is determined by two factors: attitude towards the behaviour and subjective norm or perceived social pressure to perform (or not perform) the behaviour. Attitude is the product of a set of salient beliefs about the consequences of performing the

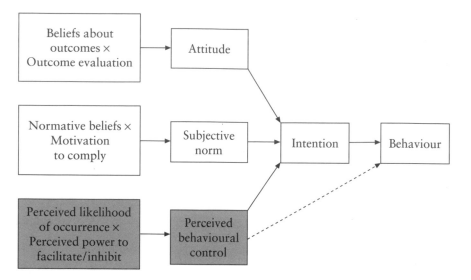

Figure 1.2   The Theories of Reasoned Action and Planned Behaviour (TPB components shown shaded in grey)

behaviour (for example 'Wearing a safety helmet would protect my head if I had an accident'), each weighted by an evaluation of the importance of each of the consequences (for example 'Protecting my head if I had an accident is good/bad'). Subjective norm is determined by the person's normative beliefs about perceived social pressure from significant others (for example 'My parents think I should wear a safety helmet') weighted by the person's motivation to comply with those others ('Generally I want to do what my parents think that I should do').

The TRA was intended to be applied to the prediction of purely volitional behaviours but, as Ajzen (1988) later argued, many behaviours are not under complete volitional control. He therefore expanded the TRA by adding the concept of perceived behavioural control, which refers to people's appraisals of their ability to perform the behaviour. According to Ajzen (1988), perceived behavioural control should predict behavioural intention and, when people's perceptions of control accurately reflect their control over behaviour, it should predict actual performance of the behaviour too. Perceived behavioural control is underpinned by control beliefs about perceptions of obstacles, impediments, skills, resources, and opportunities that may inhibit or facilitate performance of the behaviour. These may be external (for example availability of time or money) or internal (for example ability, skills).

There has been some controversy about how the construct of perceived behavioural control should be operationalized (Terry 1993; Armitage and

Conner 1999b). Ajzen and Madden (1986) first assessed it by summing the frequency of occurrence of various factors facilitating or inhibiting behavioural performance. More recently, Ajzen and his colleagues have suggested that evaluations of the power of factors likely to facilitate or inhibit performance of the behaviour should be weighted by their frequency of occurrence (Ajzen 1991; Ajzen and Driver 1991). Other authors have suggested that perceived control over behaviour (a variant of perceived behavioural control) should be distinguished from perceived confidence in one's own ability to perform the behaviour (self-efficacy) and that both constructs should be measured (Terry 1993; Terry and O'Leary 1995; Conner and Armitage 1998; Armitage and Conner 1999a; Povey *et al.* 2000; Abraham, Wight and Scott, Chapter 2 in this volume).

Both the TRA and the TPB have attracted enormous attention from social psychologists interested in identifying beliefs underpinning health behaviours that may be amenable to change, and the models have received extensive support: see Sheppard *et al.* (1988) and Van den Putte (1993) for reviews of the TRA; Ajzen (1991), Conner and Sparks (1996), Godin and Kok (1996), Conner and Armitage (1998), Ajzen and Fishbein (2000), Armitage and Conner (2000) and Armitage and Conner (in press) for reviews of the TPB; and Sheeran and Taylor (1999) and Albarracín *et al.* (2001) for meta-analyses and comparisons of the TRA and TPB. Godin and Kok (1996), in a review of the TPB's application to *health* behaviours, found that components of the TPB explain on average 41 per cent of the variance in intention; in a review of a wider range of behaviours, Armitage and Conner (in press) found that the TPB accounted for 39 per cent of the variance.

The prediction of *behaviour* from TRA and TPB variables is less impressive. Godin and Kok's (1996) review found that TPB constructs accounted for only 31 per cent of the variance in behaviour in prospective studies, while Armitage and Conner (in press) found a figure of 27 per cent. The work of other researchers has generally confirmed these findings (Sheppard *et al.* 1988; Randall and Wolff 1994; Sheeran and Orbell 1998; Sutton 1998). Since the large amount of unexplained variance is unlikely to be due to measurement error, this suggests a role for other variables.

One of the central tenets of the TRA and TPB has been that the models are 'sufficient' – that is, that variables external to the models fail to account for additional variance in intentions or behavioural performance once the effects of the models' components have been taken into account. A number of researchers have attempted to challenge this assumption and to increase the predictive power of the model by including additional variables. Many of these have been described by Eagly and Chaiken (1993: 177–93) and Manstead and Parker (1995). A number of the constructs are hypothesized to account for variance in behavioural intention over and above what is accounted for by the TPB or TRA. They include personal/moral norm or perceived moral obligation (Beck and Ajzen 1991; Boyd and Wandersman

1991; Sparks 1994; Parker *et al.* 1995; Conner and McMillan 1999; Evans and Norman, Chapter 9 in this volume); anticipated regret (Parker *et al.* 1995 and Parker, Chapter 8 in this volume; Evans and Norman, Chapter 9); anticipated affect (Van der Pligt and de Vries 1998; Bish *et al.* 2000); and affective evaluations of behaviour (Manstead and Parker 1995). A further construct, self-identity (see Evans and Norman, Chapter 9), has been proposed as an extension to the TPB to improve the prediction of intention after criticisms concerning the narrow conceptualization of subjective norm and its consistently weak prediction of intention (see Van den Putte 1993; Godin and Kok 1996; Armitage *et al.* 1999; Terry *et al.* 1999). Self-identity refers to the idea that intentions are linked to identifiable societal roles and that these roles drive intention (Armitage and Conner in press). A number of studies using a version of the TPB extended to include self-identity have found support for this suggestion (Sparks and Shepherd 1992; Sparks and Guthrie 1998; Evans and Norman, Chapter 9). Yet further research has been concerned with factors that might moderate the relationship between intentions and behaviour. These include self-schemas (Sheeran and Orbell 2000a), attention control (Orbell and Sheeran 1998) and implementation intentions (Gollwitzer and Brandstätter 1997; Orbell *et al.* 1997; Sheeran and Orbell 1999; Orbell and Sheeran, Chapter 7 in this volume).

3.4 Implementation intentions

The concept of implementation intentions comes from the work of Peter Gollwitzer. Gollwitzer (1990) and Heckhausen (1991) contend that progress towards a particular goal begins with a deliberative phase in which the costs and benefits of pursuing the goal are evaluated. The *deliberative* phase results in the development of *goal intentions* or decisions whether or not to perform the behaviour. Forming a goal intention (for example 'I intend to perform X') involves committing oneself to reaching a desired outcome. Fishbein and Ajzen's (1975) Theory of Reasoned Action is similar, in that behavioural intention is seen as the immediate determinant of behaviour. However, people frequently have difficulty in translating their goals into action. Gollwitzer (1993) also proposed an *implemental* phase, in which planning when, where and how to carry out the goal-directed behaviour ('I intend to perform X whenever Y conditions are encountered') increases the likelihood that the goal will be attained. The name Gollwitzer used for these plans was *implementation intentions*.

Gollwitzer and colleagues (Gollwitzer 1993; Gollwitzer and Brandstätter 1997; Gollwitzer and Oettingen 1998; Gollwitzer and Schaal 1998; Gollwitzer 1999) have gone on to build a considerable body of empirical evidence that formulating implementation intentions furthers goal attainment. Gollwitzer and Brandstätter (1997), for example, found that students whose goal intention to write an assignment during the winter vacation was augmented by an implementation intention were more than twice as likely to submit their work on time as students who were not asked to form a plan. The implementation intention was concerned with precisely where and when the assignment would be written. Implementation intentions thus overcome the potential conflict between routes to goal realization and potential problems in translating goals into action (failing to get started, becoming distracted) by committing the individual to a specific course of action when the environmental conditions specified in their implementation intentions are encountered.

A number of studies have reported good evidence that implementation intentions can significantly increase the performance of health behaviours – including breast self-examination (Orbell *et al.* 1997), healthy eating (Verplanken and Faes 1999), attendance for cervical cancer screening (Orbell and Sheeran 1998), consumption of vitamin C pills (Sheeran and Orbell 1999) and mobility after joint replacement surgery (Orbell and Sheeran 2000). Orbell *et al.* (1997), for example, showed that women who were asked to form implementation intentions were more than twice as likely to perform breast self-examination as those who were not asked to do so. In a later intervention, Sheeran and Orbell (2000b) found that women in an experimental group who formed implementation intentions were much more likely to attend for cervical screening than women in a control group (92 per cent compared with 69 per cent), despite equal motivation. Further information about the studies is included in Chapter 7.

A question that remains for theory is *how* implementation intentions have their effect, and perhaps the most likely explanation is that they operate through *memory*. That is, they increase memory for behavioural action through the formation of plans involving anticipated environmental and contextual cues, which act as an unconscious reminder for the behaviour when they are encountered. The mechanism is probably similar to the cognitive mechanisms involved in habitual behaviour. Consistent with these suggestions, Sheeran and Orbell (2000b) found that implementation intentions mediate the relationship between intention and behaviour – suggesting that a strong memory trace is indeed formed when implementation intentions are made. A detailed account of the role of memory, and of the other possible mechanisms, is to be found in Gollwitzer (1999).

3.5 Stage models

The approaches we have discussed so far – risk perception, the Health Belief Model and the Theory of Planned Behaviour – can all be seen as *continuum* accounts of behaviour. Each takes one or more perceptions or beliefs, or perhaps sets of perceptions or beliefs, and tries to predict from their combined effect where the individual will lie on an outcome continuum such as intention or behaviour. For example, one might use behavioural beliefs, normative beliefs and control beliefs in the TPB to predict how much fat people will eat, how safely they will drive, and how likely they will be to attend for health screening. The purpose of an intervention would be to change those perceptions or beliefs in an attempt to move the person up or down the outcome continuum. Stage models, by contrast, as their name suggests, see individuals as located not on continua but at discrete, ordered *stages*, each one denoting a greater inclination to change outcome, typically behaviour, than the previous one. There are currently two main stage models in health psychology, the Transtheoretical Model (TTM) of Prochaska and DiClemente, and the Precaution Adoption Process Model (PAPM) of Weinstein (see Figure 1.3).

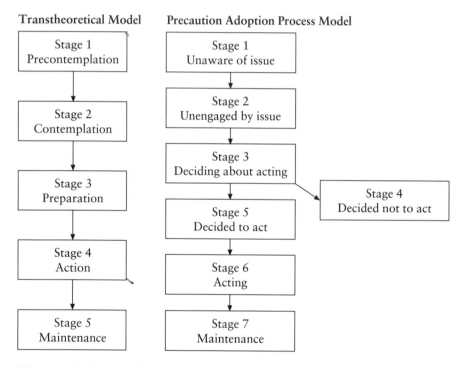

Figure 1.3   Stages of change models

The TTM proposes five stages: precontemplation (no intention of changing behaviour); contemplation (beginning to consider change, at some probably ill-defined time in the future); preparation (getting ready to change in the near future); action (engaged in change now); and maintenance (steady state of change reached). The possibility of relapse to an earlier stage is acknowledged, right back to precontemplation but not necessarily so, and the model allows that people may start the climb anew. Where an individual is to be located is defined by previous behaviour and current intentions, and the stages are seen as mutually exclusive and cannot be straddled. The model was first applied to smoking – and has been adapted by Raw (1994) as an accessible decision chart for general practitioners – but it has since been applied to a wide variety of other health behaviours too. Reviews are to be found in Prochaska *et al.* (1994), Herzog *et al.* (1999), Sutton (1999, 2000) and Velicer *et al.* (1999), and particularly accessible accounts of the model have been published in Prochaska *et al.* (1992) and Prochaska and Prochaska (1999). Evaluations of the model's constructs, methodology and findings have been published by Sutton (1996, 1997, 2001) and by Weinstein *et al.* (1998), Kraft *et al.* (1999) and Rosen (2000a, 2000b).

The PAPM is described by its author, Neil Weinstein, in Chapter 4. As its name suggests, the model is concerned with preventive or precautionary behaviour against threat. This time, there are seven stages: unaware (not aware that there is an issue or threat); unengaged (aware but not engaged); deciding about acting (considering the possibility of taking action); decided not to act; decided to act (to adopt the precaution); acting; and mainten-ance. Unlike the TTM, the PAPM thus distinguishes people who are un-aware from those who are aware but are not considering action; and it allocates those who have decided *not* to act to a stage of their own, separ-ate from those who are failing to act because they have not yet thought about the issue. Further detailed comparisons between the two models are to be found in Weinstein and Sandman (1992), Weinstein (1993) and Weinstein *et al.* (1998). The model has been applied to a variety of precau-tionary behaviours in health – including protection against osteoporosis (Blalock *et al.* 1996), hepatitis B (Hammer 1997) and radon gas (Weinstein and Sandman 1992, and Chapter 4 in this volume); and uptake of mammography (Clemow *et al.* 2000). A review is to be found in Weinstein *et al.* (1998).

The most important debate about stage models is the one suggested at the beginning of this section – whether we really do pass through stages as we move from the beginnings of awareness to behaviour, or whether 'stages' are rather points on a continuum. There are other issues too, however. Does every stage have to be visited, in a fixed order, or can a stage some-times be missed out? Do individuals located at a given stage all have to overcome the same barriers if they are to move on? What is it that triggers movement, and are particular triggers confined to one stage only or are they the same at all stages? Do the barriers and triggers cross behaviours, or do they differ by domain (taking precautions against radon or against pregnancy, for instance)? How are stage models to be tested empirically, and how are they to be used for designing and mounting interventions? Detailed accounts are to be found in Sutton (1996, 1997, 2001), Weinstein *et al.* (1998), Kraft *et al.* (1999) and Rosen (2000a, 2000b) – and in Chap-ter 4 of this volume.

4 Conclusions and future directions

To conclude the chapter, we should like to pose two questions. The first is what makes for a good intervention, and we believe the book provides a number of answers. First, and most important of all, interventions must be theory driven. Theories provide constructs, processes and hypotheses, and they point to procedures and methodologies for setting up interventions and testing their effectiveness. Without theory there is no framework or underpinning, and no progress or development. Second, interventions must tackle important health issues with identifiable associated behaviours – whether risk related, health enhancing, or any other that has serious consequences and implications. Third, processes and outcomes must be clearly defined and carefully measured, and the links between processes and procedures must be properly spelt out. Both requirements are part of having a theoretical base, and an important effect will be that the intervention can be tailored successfully to the target group or individuals. Finally, a good intervention will have implications for theory, policy, and practice, and they will be *testable* implications.

Our second question is what are the likely future directions in intervention research, and again there are strong indications in the chapters that follow. First, there will be a move towards large-scale randomized controlled trials (RCTs). Many of the interventions in the book adopt the classic 'experimental group – control group' design that is the core of the RCT, and the value of the approach for teasing out causal processes will be apparent chapter by chapter. The longer-term *added* value of full-scale RCTs will be to establish sizes of effect and reliability. Second, interventions will more frequently than now incorporate measures of *behavioural* outcome – that is, not just how much people change their perceptions, or beliefs, or intentions, but also how much they change their behaviour. Third, we must acknowledge our responsibilities to policy-makers and practitioners, and make our approaches accessible. Interventions must have an understandable theoretical base, must be easy to design, run and evaluate, and must be cost-effective. Finally, to return to our first criterion for a 'good' intervention, interventions must continue to be firmly theory driven, and we must resist the temptation to devise 'one off' attacks on behaviour based on 'common sense'. Theory provides the foundation for successful interventions, and through interventions we are able to test, and so develop, theory. From theory comes intervention and from intervention comes further theory. That, we believe, is the key theme of the book.

References

Abraham, C., Sheeran, P., Spears, R. and Abrams, D. (1992) Health beliefs and promotion of HIV-preventive intentions among teenagers: a Scottish perspective, *Health Psychology*, 11(6): 363–70.

Abraham, C., Clift, S. and Grabowski, P. (1999) Cognitive predictors of adherence to malaria prophylaxis regimens on return from a malarious region: a prospective study, *Social Science and Medicine*, 48(11): 1641–54.

Aiken, L.S., West, S.G., Woodward, C.K., Reno, R.R. and Reynolds, K.D. (1994) Increasing screening mammography in asymptomatic women: evaluation of a second-generation, theory-based program, *Health Psychology*, 13(6): 526–38.

Ajzen, I. (1988) *Attitudes, Personality and Behavior*. Milton Keynes: Open University Press.

Ajzen, I. (1991) The Theory of Planned Behavior, *Organizational Behavior and Human Decision Processes*, 50: 179–211.

Ajzen, I. and Driver, B.L. (1991) Prediction of leisure participation from behavioral, normative and control beliefs: an application of the theory of planned behavior, *Leisure Sciences*, 13: 185–204.

Ajzen, I. and Fishbein, M. (eds) (1980) *Understanding Attitudes and Predicting Social Behavior*. Englewood Cliffs, NJ: Prentice-Hall.

Ajzen, I. and Fishbein, M. (2000) Attitudes and the attitude-behavior relation: reasoned and automatic processes, in W. Stroebe and M. Hewstone (eds) *European Review of Social Psychology*, 11. Chichester: Wiley.

Ajzen, I. and Madden, T.J. (1986) Prediction of goal-directed behavior: attitudes, intention, and perceived behavioral control, *Journal of Experimental Social Psychology*, 22: 453–74.

Albarracín, D., Johnson, B.T., Fishbein, M. and Muellerleile, P.A. (2001) Theories of reasoned action and planned behavior as models of condom use: a meta-analysis, *Psychological Bulletin*, 127: 142–61.

Armitage, C.J. and Conner, M. (1999a) Distinguishing perceptions of control from self-efficacy: predicting consumption of a low fat diet using the theory of planned behavior, *Journal of Applied Social Psychology*, 29: 72–90.

Armitage, C.J. and Conner, M. (1999b) The theory of planned behaviour: assessment of predictive validity and 'perceived control', *British Journal of Social Psychology*, 38: 35–54.

Armitage, C.J. and Conner, M. (2000) Social cognition models and health behaviour: a structured review, *Psychology and Health*, 15(2): 173–89.

Armitage, C.J. and Conner, M. (in press) Efficacy of the theory of planned behaviour: a meta-analytic review, *British Journal of Social Psychology*.

Armitage, C.J., Conner, M. and Norman, P. (1999) Differential effects of mood on information processing: evidence from the theories of reasoned action and planned behaviour, *European Journal of Social Psychology*, 29(4): 419–33.

Arnold, L. and Quine, L. (1994) Predicting helmet use among schoolboy cyclists: an application of the Health Belief Model, in D.R. Rutter and L. Quine (eds) *Social Psychology and Health: European Perspectives*, 101–30. Aldershot: Avebury.

Bakker, A.B., Buunk, B.P., Siero, F.W. and van den Eijnden, R.J.J.M. (1997) Application of a modified health belief model to HIV preventive behavioral intentions among gay and bisexual men, *Psychology and Health*, 12(4): 481–92.

Beck, L. and Ajzen, I. (1991) Predicting dishonest actions using the Theory of Planned Behaviour, *Journal of Research in Personality*, 25: 285–301.

Becker, M.H. (1974) The Health Belief Model and sick role behavior, in M.H. Becker (ed.) *The Health Belief Model and Personal Health Behavior*. Thorofare, NJ: Charles B. Slack.

Becker, M.H. and Maiman, L.A. (1975) Socio-behavioural determinants of compliance with health and medical care recommendations, *Medical Care*, 13: 10–14.

Becker, M.H., Drachman, R.H. and Kirscht, J.P. (1972) Motivations as predictors of health behaviour, *Health Services Reports*, 87: 852–62.

Becker, M.H., Haefner, D.P., Kasl, S.V. et al. (1977) Selected psychosocial models and correlates of individual health-related behaviours, *Medical Care*, 15 (supplement): 27–46.

Bentler, P.M. and Speckart, G. (1979) Models of attitude–behavior relations, *Psychological Review*, 86: 452–64.

Bish, A., Sutton, S. and Golombok, S. (2000) Predicting uptake of a routine cervical smear test: a comparison of the Health Belief Model and the Theory of Planned Behaviour, *Psychology and Health*, 15: 35–50.

Blalock, S.J., DeVellis, R.F., Giorgino, K.B. et al. (1996) Osteoporosis prevention in premenopausal women: using a stage model approach to examine the predictors of behavior, *Health Psychology*, 15(2): 84–93.

Boer, H. and Seydel, E.R. (1996) Protection motivation theory, in M. Conner and P. Norman (eds) *Predicting Health Behaviour: Research and Practice with Social Cognition Models*. Buckingham: Open University Press.

Bond, G.G., Aiken, L.S. and Somerville, S.C. (1992) The health belief model and adolescents with insulin-dependent diabetes mellitus, *Health Psychology*, 11(3): 190–8.

Boyd, B. and Wandersman, A. (1991) Predicting undergraduate condom use with the Fishbein and Ajzen and the Triandis Attitude-Behaviour models: implications for public health interventions, *Journal of Applied Social Psychology*, 21(22): 1810–30.

Brenes, G.A. and Skinner, C.S. (1999) Psychological factors related to stage of mammography adoption, *Journal of Women's Health and Gender Based Medicine*, 8(10): 1313–21.

Brown, C.M. and Segal, R. (1996) The effects of health and treatment perceptions on the use of prescribed medication and home remedies among African American and White American hypertensives, *Social Science and Medicine*, 43(6): 903–17.

Budd, R.J., Hughes, I.C.T. and Smith, J.A. (1996) Health beliefs and compliance with antipsychotic medication, *British Journal of Clinical Psychology*, 35(3): 393–7.

Burger, J.M. and Palmer, M.L. (1992) Changes in and generalization of unrealistic optimism following experiences with stressful events: reactions to the 1989 California earthquake, *Personality and Social Psychology*, 18(1): 39–43.

Calnan, M. (1984) The health belief model and participation in programmes for the early detection of breast cancer: a comparative analysis, *Social Science and Medicine*, 19: 823–30.

Champion, V.L. (1984) Instrument development for Health Belief Model constructs, *Advances in Nursing Science*, 6: 73–85.

Champion, V.L. (1990) Breast self-examination in women 35 and older: a prospective study, *Journal of Behavioral Medicine*, 13(6): 523–38.

Champion, V.L. and Miller, T. (1996) Predicting mammography utilization through model generation, *Psychology, Health and Medicine*, 1(3): 273–83.

Clemow, L., Costanza, M.E., Haddad, W.P. et al. (2000) Underutilizers of mammography screening today: characteristics of women planning, undecided about, and not planning a mammogram, *Annals of Behavioral Medicine*, 22(1): 80–8.

Conner, M. and Armitage, C.J. (1998) Extending the theory of planned behavior: a review and avenues for further research, *Journal of Applied Social Psychology*, 28(15): 1429–64.

Conner, M. and McMillan, B. (1999) Interaction effects in the theory of planned behaviour: studying cannabis use, *British Journal of Social Psychology*, 38(2): 195–222.

Conner, M. and Norman, P. (1994) Comparing the Health Belief Model and the Theory of Planned Behaviour in health screening, in D.R. Rutter and L. Quine (eds) *Social Psychology and Health: European Perspectives*. Aldershot: Avebury.

Conner, M. and Norman, P. (eds) (1996) *Predicting Health Behaviour: Research and Practice with Social Cognition Models*. Buckingham: Open University Press.

Conner, M. and Sparks, P. (1996) The theory of planned behaviour and health behaviours, in M. Conner and P. Norman (eds) *Predicting Health Behaviour: Research and Practice with Social Cognition Models*. Buckingham: Open University Press.

Corwyn, R.F. and Benda, B.B. (1999) Examination of an integrated theoretical model of exercise behavior, *American Journal of Health Behavior*, 23(5): 381–92.

Dolinski, D., Gromski, W. and Zawisza, E. (1987) Unrealistic pessimism, *Journal of Social Psychology*, 127(5): 511–16.

Dracup, K., Moser, D.K., Eisenberg, M. *et al.* (1995) Causes of delay in seeking treatment for heart attack symptoms, *Social Science and Medicine*, 40(3): 379–92.

Eagly, A.H. and Chaiken, S. (1993) *The Psychology of Attitudes*. New York: Harcourt Brace and Jovanovich.

Fischera, S.D. and Frank, D.I. (1994) The Health Belief Model as a predictor of mammography screening, *Health Values: The Journal of Health Behavior, Education and Promotion*, 18(4): 3–9.

Fishbein, M. and Ajzen, I. (1975) *Belief, Attitude, Intention and Behavior: An Introduction to Theory and Research*. Reading, MA: Addison-Wesley.

Friedman, L.C., Nelson, D.V., Webb, J.A. *et al.* (1994) Dispositional optimism, self-efficacy, and health beliefs as predictors of breast self-examination, *American Journal of Preventive Medicine*, 10(3): 130–5.

Gerrard, M., Gibbons, F.X. and Bushman, B.J. (1996) Relation between perceived vulnerability to HIV and precautionary sexual behaviour, *Psychology Bulletin*, 119(1): 390–409.

Godin, G. and Kok, G. (1996) The Theory of Planned Behavior: a review of its applications to health-related behaviors, *American Journal of Health Promotion*, 11(2): 87–98.

Gollwitzer, P.M. (1990) Action phases and mind-sets, in E.T. Higgins and R.M. Sorrentino (eds) *Handbook of Motivation and Cognition: Foundations of Social Behavior*, 2, 53–92. New York: Guilford.

Gollwitzer, P.M. (1993) Goal achievement: the role of intentions, in W. Stroebe and M. Hewstone (eds) *European Review of Social Psychology*, 4. Chichester: Wiley.

Gollwitzer, P.M. (1999) Implementation intentions: strong effects of simple plans, *American Psychologist*, 54(7): 493–503.

Gollwitzer, P.M. and Brandstätter, V. (1997) Implementation intentions and effective goal pursuit, *Journal of Personality and Social Psychology*, 73(1): 186–99.

Gollwitzer, P.M. and Oettingen, G. (1998) The emergence and implementation of health goals, *Psychology and Health*, 13(4): 687–715.

Gollwitzer, P.M. and Schaal, B. (1998) Metacognition in action: the importance of implementation intentions, *Personality and Social Psychology Review*, 2(2): 124–36.

Haefner, D.P. and Kirscht, L.P. (1970) Motivational and behavioural effects of modifying health beliefs, *Public Health Reports*, 85: 478–84.

Hammer, G.P. (1997) Hepatitis B vaccine acceptance among nursing home workers. Unpublished dissertation, Department of Health Policy and Management, Johns Hopkins University, Baltimore, MD.

Harris, P. (1996) Sufficient grounds for optimism? The relationship between perceived controllability and optimistic bias, *Journal of Social and Clinical Psychology*, 15(1): 9–52.

Harris, P. and Middleton, W. (1994) The illusion of control and optimism about health: on being less at risk but no more in control than others, *British Journal of Social Psychology*, 33: 369–86.

Harrison, J.A., Mullen, P.D. and Green, L.W. (1992) A meta-analysis of studies of the Health Belief Model with adults, *Health Education Research*, 7: 107–16.

Heckhausen, H. (1991) *Motivation and Action*. Berlin: Springer-Verlag.

Herzog, T.A., Abrams, D.B., Emmons, K.M., Linnan, L.A. and Shadel, W.G. (1999) Do processes of change predict smoking stage movements? A prospective analysis of the transtheoretical model, *Health Psychology*, 18(4): 369–75.

Hill, D., Gardner, G. and Rassaby, J. (1985) Factors predisposing women to take precautions against breast and cervix cancer, *Journal of Applied Social Psychology*, 15: 59–79.

Hoorens, V. (1994) Unrealistic optimism in health and safety risks, in D.R. Rutter and L. Quine (eds) *Social Psychology and Health: European Perspectives*. Aldershot: Avebury.

Hoorens, V. (1996) Sufficient grounds for optimism? The relationship between perceived controllability and optimistic bias, *Journal of Social and Clinical Psychology*, 15(1): 9–52.

Hughes, I., Hill, B. and Budd, R. (1997) Compliance with antipsychotic medication: from theory to practice, *Journal of Mental Health UK*, 6(5): 473–89.

Janz, N. and Becker, M.H. (1984) The health belief model: a decade later, *Health Education Quarterly*, 11: 1–47.

King, J.B. (1982) The impact of patients' perceptions of high blood pressure on attendance at screening: an extension of the health belief model, *Social Science and Medicine*, 16: 1079–91.

Kraft, P., Sutton, S.R. and Reynolds, H.M. (1999) The transtheoretical model of behaviour change: are the stages qualitatively different?, *Psychology and Health*, 14(3): 433–50.

Kreuter, M.W. and Strecher, V.J. (1995) Changing inaccurate perceptions of health risk: results from a randomized trial, *Health Psychology*, 14(1): 56–63.

Lau, R.R., Hartman, K.A. and Ware, J.E. (1986) Health as a value: methodological and theoretical considerations, *Health Psychology*, 5: 25–43.

Leenaars, P.E., Rombouts, R. and Kok, G. (1993) Seeking medical care for a sexually transmitted disease: determinants of delay-behavior, *Psychology and Health*, 8(1): 17–32.

Lux, K.M. and Petosa, R. (1994) Using the health belief model to predict safer sex intentions of incarcerated youth, *Health Education Quarterly*, 21(4): 487–97.

McKenna, F.P. (1993) It won't happen to me: unrealistic optimism or illusion of control?, *British Journal of Psychology*, 84: 39–50.

McKenna, F.P. and Albery, I. (2001) Does unrealistic optimism change following a negative experience?, *Journal of Applied Social Psychology*, 31(6): 1146–57.

McKenna, F.P. and Myers, L.B. (1997) Can accountability reduce or reverse existing illusory self assessments?, *British Journal of Psychology*, 88: 39–51.

Manstead, A.S.R. and Parker, D. (1995) Evaluating and extending the theory of planned behaviour, in W. Stroebe and M. Hewstone (eds) *European Review of Social Psychology*, 6. Chichester: Wiley.

Melnyk, K.A.M. (1988) Barriers: a critical review of recent literature, *Nursing Research*, 37: 196–201.

Millar, M.G. (1997) The effects of emotion on breast self-examination: another look at the Health Belief Model, *Social Behavior and Personality*, 25(3): 223–32.

Myers, L.B. and Reynolds, R. (2000) How optimistic are repressors? The relationship between repressive coping, controllability, self-esteem and optimism for health-related events, *Psychology and Health*, 15: 667–88.

Nageotte, C., Sullivan, G., Duan, N. and Camp, P.L. (1997) Medication compliance among the seriously mentally ill in a public mental health system, *Social Psychiatry and Psychiatric Epidemiology*, 32(2): 49–56.

Norman, P. and Conner, M. (1993) The role of social cognition models in predicting attendance at health checks, *Psychology and Health*, 8(6): 447–62.

Norman, P. and Fitter, M. (1989) Intentions to attend a health screening appointment: some implications for general practice, *Counselling Psychology Quarterly*, 2: 261–72.

Oliver, R.L. and Berger, P.K. (1979) A path-analysis of preventive health care decision models, *Journal of Consumer Research*, 6: 113–22.

Orbell, S. and Sheeran, P. (1998) 'Inclined abstainers': a problem for predicting health-related behaviour, *British Journal of Social Psychology*, 37: 151–65.

Orbell, S. and Sheeran, P. (2000) Motivational and volitional processes in action initiation: a field study of the role of implementation intentions, *Journal of Applied Social Psychology*, 30: 780–97.

Orbell, S., Crombie, I. and Johnston, G. (1996) Social cognition and social structure in the prediction of cervical screening uptake, *British Journal of Health Psychology*, 1(1): 35–50.

Orbell, S., Hodgkins, S. and Sheeran, P. (1997) Implementation intentions and the theory of planned behavior, *Personality and Social Psychology Bulletin*, 23(9): 945–54.

Otten, W. and Van der Pligt, J. (1992) Risk and behavior: the mediating role of risk appraisal, *Acta Psychologica*, 80: 325–46.

Parker, D., Manstead, A.S.R. and Stradling, S.G. (1995) Extending the theory of planned behaviour: the role of personal norm, *British Journal of Social Psychology*, 34: 127–37.

Perloff, L.S. and Fetzer, B.K. (1986) Self–other judgements and perceived vulnerability to victimization, *Journal of Personality and Social Psychology*, 50(3): 502–10.

Petosa, R. and Jackson, K. (1991) Using the health belief model to predict safer sex intentions among adolescents, *Health Education Quarterly*, 18(4): 463–76.

Povey, R., Conner, M., Sparks, P., James, R. and Shepherd, R. (2000) Application of the Theory of Planned Behaviour to two dietary behaviours: roles of perceived control and self-efficacy, *British Journal of Health Psychology*, 5(2): 121–39.

Prentice-Dunn, S. and Rogers, R.W. (1986) Protection motivation theory and preventive health: beyond the health belief model, *Health Education Research*, 1(3): 153–61.

Prochaska, J.O. and Prochaska, J.M. (1999) Why don't continents move? Why don't people change?, *Journal of Psychotherapy Integration*, 9(1): 83–102.

Prochaska, J.O., DiClemente, C.C. and Norcross, J.C. (1992) In search of how people change: applications to addictive behaviors, *American Psychologist*, 47(9): 1102–14.

Prochaska, J.O., Redding, C.A., Harlow, L.L., Rossi, J.S. and Velicer, W.F. (1994) The Transtheoretical Model of Change and HIV prevention: a review, *Health Education Quarterly*, 21(4): 471–86.

Quine, L., Rutter, D.R. and Arnold, L. (1998) Predicting and understanding safety helmet use among schoolboy cyclists: a comparison of the Theory of Planned Behaviour and the Health Belief Model, *Psychology and Health*, 13: 251–69.

Randall, D.M. and Wolff, J.A. (1994) The time interval in the intention-behaviour relationship: meta-analysis, *British Journal of Social Psychology*, 33: 405–18.

Raw, M. (1994) *How to Explain to Smokers that it is Worth Stopping*. London: Health Education Authority.

Rogers, R.W. (1975) A protection motivation theory of fear appeals and attitude change, *Journal of Psychology*, 91: 93–114.

Rogers, R.W. (1985) Attitude change and information integration in fear appeals, *Psychological Reports*, 56: 179–82.

Rosen, C.S. (2000a) Integrating stage and continuum models to explain processing of exercise messages and exercise initiation among sedentary college students, *Health Psychology*, 19(2): 172–80.

Rosen, C.S. (2000b) Is the sequencing of change processes by stage consistent across health problems? A meta-analysis, *Health Psychology*, 19(6): 593–604.

Rosenstock, I.M. (1966) Why people use health services, *Milbank Memorial Fund Quarterly*, 44: 94–124.

Rosenstock, I.M. (1974a) The Health Belief Model and preventive health behavior, *Health Education Monographs*, 2: 354–86.

Rosenstock, I.M. (1974b) Historical origins of the Health Belief Model, in M.H. Becker (ed.) *The Health Belief Model and Personal Health Behavior*. Thorofare, NJ: Charles B. Slack.

Rutledge, D.N. (1987) Factors related to women's practice of breast self-examination, *Nursing Research*, 36: 117–21.

Savage, S.A. and Clarke, V.A. (1996) Factors associated with screening mammography and breast self-examination, *Health Education Research*, 11(4): 409–21.

Schwarzer, R. (1992) Self-efficacy in the adoption and maintenance of health behaviors: theoretical approaches and a new model, in R. Schwarzer (ed.) *Self-efficacy: Thought Control of Action*. Washington, DC: Hemisphere.

Schwarzer, R. (1994) Optimism, vulnerability, and self-beliefs as health-related cognitions: a systematic overview, *Psychology and Health*, 9: 161–80.

Schwarzer, R. (1999) Self-regulatory processes in the adoption and maintenance of health behaviors: the role of optimism, goals, and threats, *Journal of Health Psychology*, 4(2): 115–27.

Schwarzer, R. and Fuchs, R. (1996) Self-efficacy and health behaviours, in M. Conner and P. Norman (eds) *Predicting Health Behaviour*. Buckingham: Open University Press.

Sheeran, P. and Abraham, C. (1996) The health belief model, in M. Conner and P. Norman (eds) *Predicting Health Behaviour*. Buckingham: Open University Press.

Sheeran, P. and Orbell, S. (1998) Do intentions predict condom use? Meta-analysis and examination of six moderator variables, *British Journal of Social Psychology*, 37: 231–50.

Sheeran, P. and Orbell, S. (1999) Implementation intentions and repeated behaviour: augmenting the predictive validity of the theory of planned behaviour, *European Journal of Social Psychology*, 29: 349–69.

Sheeran, P. and Orbell, S. (2000a) Self-schemas and the theory of planned behaviour, *European Journal of Social Psychology*, 30: 533–50.

Sheeran, P. and Orbell, S. (2000b) Using implementation intentions to increase attendance for cervical cancer screening, *Health Psychology*, 19(3): 283–9.

Sheeran, P. and Taylor, S. (1999) Predicting intentions to use condoms: a meta-analysis and comparison of the theories of reasoned action and planned behavior, *Journal of Applied Social Psychology*, 29(8): 1624–75.

Sheppard, B.H., Hartwick, J. and Warshaw, P.R. (1988) The Theory of Reasoned Action: a meta-analysis of past research with recommendations for modifications and future research, *Journal of Consumer Research*, 15: 325–39.

Simon, P.M., Morse, E.V., Balson, P.M., Osofsky, H.J. and Gaumer, H.R. (1993) Barriers to human immunodeficiency virus related risk reduction among male street prostitutes, *Health Education Quarterly*, 20: 261–73.

Sparks, P. (1994) Food choice and health: applying, assessing, and extending the Theory of Planned Behaviour, in D.R. Rutter and L. Quine (eds) *Social Psychology and Health: European Perspectives*. Aldershot: Avebury.

Sparks, P. and Guthrie, C.A. (1998) Self-identity and the theory of planned behavior: a useful addition or an unhelpful artifice?, *Journal of Applied Social Psychology*, 28(15): 1393–410.

Sparks, P. and Shepherd, R. (1992) Self-identity and the theory of planned behavior: assessing the role of identification with green consumerism, *Social Psychology Quarterly*, 55: 388–99.

Stapel, D.A. and Velthuijsen, A.S. (1996) 'Just as if it happened to me': the impact of vivid and self-relevant information on risk judgments, *Journal of Social and Clinical Psychology*, 15(1): 102–19.

Steers, W.N., Elliot, E., Nemiro, J., Ditman, D. and Oskamp, S. (1996) Health beliefs as predictors of HIV-preventive behavior and ethnic differences in prediction, *Journal of Social Psychology*, 136(1): 99–110.

Sutton, S. (1996) Can 'stages of change' provide guidance in the treatment of addictions? A critical examination of Prochaska and DiClemente's model, in G.E. Edwards and C. Dare (eds) *Psychotherapy, Psychological Treatments and the Addictions*. Cambridge: Cambridge University Press.

Sutton, S. (1997) Theory of planned behaviour, in A. Baum, S. Newman, J. Weinman, R. West and C. McManus (eds) *Cambridge Handbook of Psychology, Health and Medicine*. Cambridge: Cambridge University Press.

Sutton, S. (1998) Predicting and explaining intentions and behavior: how well are we doing? *Journal of Applied Social Psychology*, 28(15): 1317–38.

Sutton, S. (1999) Project MATCH and the stages of change, *Addiction*, 94(1): 47–8.

Sutton, S. (2000) A critical review of the transtheoretical model applied to smoking cessation, in P. Norman, C. Abraham and M. Conner (eds) *Understanding and Changing Health Behaviour: From Health Beliefs to Self-Regulation*. Amsterdam: Harwood.

Sutton, S. (2001) Back to the drawing board? A review of applications of the transtheoretical model to substance use, *Addiction*, 96(1): 175–86.

Svenson, O., Fischhoff, B. and MacGregor, D. (1985) Perceived driving safety and seatbelt usage, *Accident Analysis and Prevention*, 17: 119–33.

Taylor, S.E. and Armor, D.A. (1996) Positive illusions and coping with adversity, *Journal of Personality*, 64(4): 873–98.

Terry, D.J. (1993) Self-efficacy expectancies and the theory of reasoned action, in D.J. Terry, C. Gallois and M. McCamish (eds) *The Theory of Reasoned Action: Its Application to AIDS-related Behavior*. Oxford: Pergamon.

Terry, D.J. and O'Leary, J.E. (1995) The theory of planned behaviour: the effects of perceived behavioural control and self-efficacy, *British Journal of Social Psychology*, 34: 199–220.

Terry, D.J., Hogg, M.A. and White, K.M. (1999) The theory of planned behaviour: self-identity, social identity and group norms, *British Journal of Social Psychology*, 38(3): 225–44.

Van den Putte, B. (1993) On the theory of reasoned action. Unpublished doctoral dissertation, University of Amsterdam.

Van der Pligt, J. (1991) Risk perception, unrealistic optimism, and AIDS-prevention behavior, *Nederlands Tijdschrift voor de Psychologie en haar Grensgebieden*, 46: 228–37.

Van der Pligt, J. (1994) Risk appraisal and health behaviour, in D.R. Rutter and L. Quine (eds) *Social Psychology and Health: European Perspectives*. Aldershot: Avebury.

Van der Pligt, J. (1998) Perceived risk and vulnerability as predictors of precautionary behaviour, *British Journal of Health Psychology*, 3(1): 1–14.

Van der Pligt, J. and de Vries, N.K. (1998) Expectancy-value models of health behavior: the role of salience and anticipated affect, *Psychology and Health*, 13: 289–305.

Van der Velde, F.W. and van der Pligt, J. (1991) AIDS-related health behavior: coping, protection motivation and previous behavior, *Journal of Behavioral Medicine*, 14: 429–52.

Van der Velde, F.W., Hooijkaas, C. and van der Pligt, J. (1992) Risk perception and behavior: pessimism, realism, and optimism about AIDS-related health behavior, *Psychology and Health*, 6: 23–8.

Velicer, W.F., Norman, G.J., Fava, J.L. and Prochaska, J.O. (1999) Testing 40 predictions from the transtheoretical model, *Addictive Behaviours*, 24(4): 455–69.

Verplanken, B. and Faes, S. (1999) Good intentions, bad habits, and effects of forming implementation intentions on healthy eating, *European Journal of Social Psychology*, 29(5–6): 591–604.

Wallston, K.A. and Wallston, B.S. (1981) Health locus of control scales, in H.M. Lefcourt (ed.) *Research with the Locus of Control Constant I: Assessment Methods*. New York: Academic Press.

Walter, H.J., Vaughan, R.D., Gladis, M.M. *et al.* (1993) Factors associated with AIDS-related behavioral intentions among high school students in an AIDS epicenter, *Health Education Quarterly*, 20(3): 409–20.

Weinstein, N.D. (1980) Unrealistic optimism about future life events, *Journal of Personality and Social Psychology*, 39(5): 806–20.

Weinstein, N.D. (1982) Unrealistic optimism about susceptibility to health problems, *Journal of Behavioral Medicine*, 5(4): 441–60.

Weinstein, N.D. (1983) Reducing unrealistic optimism about illness susceptibility, *Health Psychology*, 2(1): 11–20.

Weinstein, N.D. (1984) Why it won't happen to me: perceptions of risk factors and susceptibility, *Health Psychology*, 3(5): 431–57.

Weinstein, N.D. (1987) Unrealistic optimism about susceptibility to health problems: conclusions from a community-wide sample, *Journal of Behavioral Medicine*, 10: 481–500.

Weinstein, N.D. (1988) The precaution adoption process, *Health Psychology*, 7(4): 355–86.

Weinstein, N.D. (1989) Optimistic bias about personal risks, *Science*, 246: 1232–3.

Weinstein, N.D. (1993) Testing four competing theories of health-protective behaviour, *Health Psychology*, 12(4): 324–33.

Weinstein, N.D. and Klein, W.M. (1995) Resistance of personal risk perceptions to debiasing interventions, *Health Psychology*, 14(2): 132–40.

Weinstein, N.D. and Klein, W.M. (1996) Unrealistic optimism: present and future, *Journal of Social and Clinical Psychology*, 15(1): 1–8.

Weinstein, N.D. and Nicolich, M. (1993) Correct and incorrect interpretations of correlations between risk perceptions and risk behaviours, *Health Psychology*, 12(3): 235–45.

Weinstein, N.D. and Sandman, P.M. (1992) A model of the precaution adoption process: evidence from home radon testing, *Health Psychology*, 11(3): 170–80.

Weinstein, N.D., Rothman, A.J. and Sutton, S.R. (1998) Stage theories of health behavior: conceptual and methodological issues, *Health Psychology*, 17(3): 290–9.

Weinstein, N.D., Sandman, P.M. and Roberts, N.E. (1990) Determinants of self-protective behavior: home radon testing, *Journal of Applied Social Psychology*, 20: 783–801.

Witte, K., Stokols, D., Ituarte, P. and Schneider, M. (1993) Testing the Health Belief Model in a field study to promote bicycle safety helmets, *Communication Research*, 20: 564–86.

Wyper, M.A. (1990) Breast self-examination and the Health Belief Model: variations on a theme, *Research in Nursing and Health*, 13: 421–8.

2	CHARLES ABRAHAM, DANIEL WIGHT AND SUE SCOTT

ENCOURAGING SAFER-SEX BEHAVIOURS: DEVELOPMENT OF THE SHARE SEX EDUCATION PROGRAMME

This chapter describes the development of a teacher-led, school-based sex education programme, currently undergoing a randomized controlled trial in the south-east of Scotland. The theoretical basis of the intervention is outlined and some of the practical difficulties encountered in translating theoretical ideas into potentially effective classroom sessions are discussed. We conclude that it is possible to develop a potentially effective, research-based, teacher-led sex education programme that could be widely disseminated. However, we emphasize that theoretical insights must be sensitively translated into sessions taking account of classroom culture and the needs and skills of teachers. We also highlight some potential difficulties involved in integrating research and practice in this area.

1 Encouraging safer-sex behaviours

1.1 Do we need research-based sex education in schools?

The spread of the human immunodeficiency virus (HIV) highlighted the biological threats inherent in sexual activity, and research into sexual behaviour has further underlined the need for intervention in this area. The reported median age at first intercourse is falling in the UK. A national survey conducted in the early 1990s estimated that 19 per cent of 16–19-year-old women and 28 per cent of 16–19-year-old men reported sexual intercourse before 16 (Johnson *et al.* 1994). More recently, a survey of more than 7500 13–14 year olds in Scotland found that 15 per cent of girls and 18 per cent of boys reported heterosexual intercourse by the age of 14

(Wight *et al.* 2000). More than half of the reported instances of first intercourse were unplanned in this sample and only 40 per cent were judged to have happened at the right time. For both first and last intercourse approximately 60 per cent of boys and girls alike reported that condoms were 'used throughout', while 21 per cent reported using some other form of contraception. In addition, 75 per cent of these 13–14-year-olds reported experience of 'kissing using tongues', indicating a widespread involvement in romantic/sexual encounters.

It is unsurprising that teenagers seek romantic and sexual involvement in a media-permeated culture in which the commercialization of sexual semiotics is commonplace, even in media designed for teenage consumption (for example McRobbie 1996; Wellings 1996). It is, however, of concern that teenagers may not be adequately prepared for these experiences, which may lead to poorly planned sexual encounters, relationship breakdown, sexually transmitted infections (STIs) and unwanted pregnancies (for example Bury 1984; Johnson *et al.* 1994; Wight 1994). For example, more than 40,000 terminations are performed on teenagers in the UK each year and chlamydia and associated pelvic inflammatory disease are increasing among young women (Royal College of Obstetricians and Gynaecologists (RCOG) 1991; Health Education Authority 1994; Scottish Needs Assessment Programme 1994).

Such concerns, and particularly the fear of a devastating HIV epidemic, have prompted rapid and widespread investment in safer-sex promotion in the UK and elsewhere (for example Fisher and Fisher 1992; Berridge and Strong 1993). This admirable response has not, unfortunately, allowed time to develop theoretically based and carefully tested educational programmes. For example, the first UK mass media campaign relied on a 'Don't die of ignorance' slogan accompanied by images of tombstones. Yet prior psychological findings had demonstrated that fear appeals are most likely to influence behaviour when they are accompanied by clear instructions on how to take preventive action (Leventhal 1970) and previous evaluations had suggested that fear-arousing anti-heroin campaigns were regarded as unrealistic by their target audience (Coggans *et al.* 1991).

Predictably, few of these early campaigns were found to change sexual behaviour (for example Sherr 1987; Ross *et al.* 1990) and, in a comprehensive review, Fisher and Fisher (1992) found few effective HIV-preventive interventions. Fisher and Fisher (1992: 463) concluded that this was because 'AIDS reduction efforts that have been based on formal conceptualisations of any kind are exceedingly rare'. They also noted that effective interventions were 'conceptually-based' and provided 'AIDS-risk information, motivation and behavioural skills' (1992: 463). Similarly, in a review of school-based sex education programmes, Kirby *et al.* (1994) identified the use of social cognitive theory (Bandura 1986) in the intervention design as one of the factors that distinguished effective from ineffective curricula.

In a review of interventions designed for young people, Oakley *et al.* (1995) judged 12 of 65 identified outcome-evaluation studies to be methodologically sound but found only 2 that showed clear evidence of a subsequent change in young people's sexual behaviour. One of these, a safer-sex intervention for teenage runaways, found an increase in reported condom use and decreased risk behaviour (Rotheram-Borus *et al.* 1991), while the other, a programme designed to promote sexual abstinence, *increased* sexual initiation among young men in the intervention condition (Christopher and Roosa 1991). It should be noted, however, that some programmes that appear to have been effective were excluded from Oakley *et al.*'s (1995) review because their evaluation reports did not meet exacting methodological criteria (for example Jemmott *et al.* 1992; Walter and Vaughan 1993). Moreover, the most reliable evidence indicates that school sex education does *not* increase sexual activity or pregnancy rates (National Health Service Centre for Reviews and Dissemination 1997).

More recent interventions have used psychological findings on the antecedents of behaviour change to define learning objectives and change targets. Early evaluations are encouraging. For example, Schaalma *et al.* (1996) found that an HIV-preventive school curriculum based on social cognition models was more effective in changing teenagers' cognitions than standard Dutch sex education. In particular, the intervention had a significant effect on the behaviour of students reporting risk-taking behaviour at baseline. For example, while 45 per cent of those reporting inconsistent condom use with a sexual partner at baseline continued to report sexual risk-taking after receiving standard Dutch sex education, only 36 per cent of those receiving the theory-based programme continued to report risk behaviour. Similarly, Bryan *et al.* (1996) evaluated a single-session intervention based on social cognitive models to promote condom use among college women. Results showed that significantly greater numbers of women in the intervention group reported condom use during last intercourse at both six-week (68 per cent vs 43 per cent) and six-month follow-ups (68 per cent vs 49 per cent). In a meta-analysis of twelve controlled trials of HIV-preventive interventions based on social cognitive theory, Kalichman *et al.* (1996) reported significant overall effect sizes equalling or exceeding in magnitude those achieved by interventions routinely employed in other areas of health care.

Such findings indicate that safer-sex interventions based on psychological insights into cognitive and behavioural regulation are most likely to be effective, and suggests that information provision alone is inadequate (Abraham *et al.* 1998b). Undoubtedly, the prevention of sexually transmitted infections depends on disseminating a good understanding of sexual practices and associated transmission risks. However, the regulation of sexual behaviour depends on cognitive and social skills required to manage and negotiate sexual interaction (for example Miller *et al.* 1993). Evidence of sexual coercion (Biglan *et al.* 1995), widespread anxiety (Wight 1994) and regretted experiences (Johnson *et al.* 1994) suggests that current provision is failing to empower young people to manage the social and emotional realities of romantic and sexual relationships. In the UK the need to address this problem is gaining support among public health policy makers. For example, in 1992 specific sexual health targets were set in the UK government's *Health of the Nation* strategy document (Department of Health 1992) and a more recent report on teenage pregnancy by the Social Exclusion Unit (1999) recommended educational interventions designed to delay first sexual intercourse.

1.2 The SHARE programme

The SHARE project (Sexual Health and Relationships: Safe Happy and Responsible) began with research into sex education in schools in eastern Scotland (Wight and Scott 1994). This included a needs assessment as well as exploration of practical opportunities for implementating an innovative programme. The results prompted and shaped the development of a teacher-delivered sex education programme which aims to

- reduce the incidence of unsafe sex
- improve the quality of young people's romantic and sexual relationships
- reduce the rate of unwanted pregnancies.

The development of the programme was based on four principles, namely, that the programme should

- be theoretically based and apply findings from recent social science research into young people's sexuality
- draw upon the best existing sex education materials and practice
- be sufficiently standardized to allow rigorous evaluation
- be readily replicable and sustainable within existing school environments.

The resulting programme includes an integral five-day teacher training course and a teachers' resource pack of twenty sessions. It is designed to be delivered over two school years to those below the minimum school leaving age, 16. This allows the programme to be delivered to almost all young people at state-supported, secondary-level schools and, unlike most service provision and community education, ensures that as many young men as women can be reached (Abraham and Wight 1996). Younger children were not targeted because it was thought that too few would consider the programme personally relevant and because this would have limited the content deemed acceptable by education authorities and parents.

The teacher training course and resource pack were piloted in four Scottish schools with nine teachers and seventeen classes. The training was evaluated through participant observation, participants' self completed questionnaires and semi-structured interviews. The programme was evaluated using a brief teacher questionnaire for each session, semi-structured interviews with teachers and pupils, group discussions with pupils, and observation of sessions (Wight and Scott 1996). The SHARE team also received advice and comment from five UK sex education experts as well as leading researchers involved in the development and evaluation of previous classroom-based programmes (for example Kirby *et al.* 1994; Mellanby *et al.* 1995; Schaalma *et al.* 1996). The research and feedback together resulted in substantial changes to pilot materials, illustrating the importance of an iterative approach to development, in which practical constraints are addressed in the design and piloting stage (Bartholomew *et al.* 1998).

The revised training course and programme were piloted in a further 4 schools. This second pilot involved 15 teachers and 23 classes and employed similar methods to those used before, but included a largely open-ended self-complete questionnaire, which was administered to 115 pupils. Smaller changes were made as a result of this second pilot and a randomized controlled trial of the full programme began in 1996.

2 Theoretical perspective: symbolic interactionism and script theory

In accordance with our first development principle, design work drew upon analyses of young people's sexual behaviour employing symbolic interactionism and script theory (for example Gagnon and Simon 1974), phenomenology (for example Bloor *et al.* 1993), analyses of power relations in heterosexual interactions (Holland *et al.* 1998) and research demonstrating the effectiveness of social cognition models in predicting young people's safer sexual behaviour (for example Catania *et al.* 1990; Fisher and Fisher 1992; Abraham and Sheeran 1994). Below we outline some of the key theoretical ideas that shaped what we did (see also Wight *et al.* 1998).

2.1 Gender and the development of heterosocial sexual identities

Symbolic interactionism proposes that identity emerges from an ongoing dialectic between one's presentation of oneself and audience views of the self (Berger and Luckmann 1966). For most young people, sexual identities are shaped primarily by interaction with same-sex peers. Feminine and masculine sexualities develop largely within the separate social worlds that boys and girls inhabit outside their families, and such separation tends to be more pronounced in working-class culture (Martin 1981). Thus, boys' and girls' valuation of themselves tends to be based on the opinions of their own sex (Gagnon and Simon 1974) and contact with the opposite sex may be most valued as a way of developing gender identity (Wight 1994).

Consequently, identities and reputations are subject to challenge or confirmation during contact with the opposite sex, and this may be especially true for young men (Wight 1994).

Sex may also contribute to the gendered divergence of sexuality development (Jackson 1982; Hawkes 1996). In many societies young men's first sexual experiences are often solitary, involving masturbation, while young women's are with a partner (Gagnon and Simon 1974). This may be due to boys' discussion of masturbation and their greater familiarity with their genitals, both because they are physically more obvious and because boys regularly handle their penises during urination. Such differences may help to explain why young men tend to focus on genital pleasure and orgasm during sex, while for young women the meaning of sex tends, to a greater extent, to be bound up with relationships.

An important task for sex education is thus to enhance young people's awareness of the homosocial (same-sex) concerns that shape their sexual identities and to reflect upon how relationships can be affected by concerns with reputation. Such education may also help young people shift from their homosocial perspective to a more heterosocial perspective. Discussing sexual issues with the opposite sex should lead to a greater understanding of and respect for opposite-gender views of romantic and sexual relationships, and is likely to desensitize the discussion of sexual topics and lead to explicit verbal scripts for such conversations. This is crucial because available evidence suggests that those who discuss contraception and condoms with their partners are more likely to use them (Gold and Berger 1983; Polit-O'Hara and Kahn 1985; Kashima *et al.* 1993). Discussion can reduce misunderstandings between inexperienced couples and disrupt non-verbal negotiation strategies that discourage explicit consideration of options during sexual interaction (Miller *et al.* 1993). The promotion of heterosocial perspectives may also encourage young men to focus on their partner rather than their social status among male peers, and young women to reflect on their relative desire for sex and romantic relationships. In short it should aim to integrate feminine and masculine perspectives of sexual relationships and to ensure that participants have had some experience of feedback and confirmation of their own sexual identities by the opposite sex.

2.2 Risk, intimacy, decision making and social control

Sex is often viewed as private and dislocated from everyday life. Yet, at the same time it is increasingly presented as a healthy leisure activity (Jackson and Scott 1996) involving acquired expertise. Young people must assimilate mixed messages from others and the media: sex is everywhere, sex is private, sex is healthy, sex is health threatening, sex is loving, sex is shameful and embarrassing, sex is risky, safer sex requires acquired expertise but everyone appears experienced and confident. Moreover, open discussion of these contradictions is problematic in many, if not most, social contexts. Thus, explicit consideration of romantic and sexual options and dispassionate evaluation of potential outcomes is rarely facilitated.

Cultural constructions of sexual activity may also inhibit individual decision making. For example, if sex is thought to be acceptable only in the context of 'being in love', or at least in a 'steady' relationship, then sexual encounters are likely to be defined by the role relations and obligations implied by these descriptions. Consequently, love and trust may become central to sexual negotiations and concerns about the risk of infection and self-protection may appear illegitimate. With reputation among friends and love at stake, personal health concerns may become secondary goals. This may make self-protective action, such as condom use, less likely because it implies an individualistic and risk-conscious approach to intimacy (Holland *et al.* 1990). Thus, encouraging young people to get to know their partners may highlight the importance of intimacy and will not necessarily encourage, and may discourage, consideration of risk and protection in sexual encounters (Scott and Freeman 1995). A dispassionate appraisal of sexual activity in the context of other life goals, and concrete advice to discuss risk and protection with potential sexual partners, are more likely to result in health care intentions taking priority during sexual negotiation.

Sexual relationships can be especially dangerous for young women, who may experience various degrees of coercion. Power, in the context of sexuality, is not simply about strength, nor can it be explained through examination of personal characteristics. It is rooted in cultural understandings that may validate men's right to have sex and to construe their sexual desires as uncontrollable (Morgan and Scott 1993). Thus, if young people are to develop a sense of agency in relation to their sexuality they need to be encouraged to be reflexive about how such perspectives affect sexual interaction. Questioning how assumptions about rights and obligations in romantic and sexual relationships are managed, and illustrating how assertive interaction control can be effected, are likely to be crucial in empowering young people to protect themselves (Abraham *et al.* 1992; Holland *et al.* 1998). Knowledge is not sufficient, nor is the desire to negotiate sexual safety. Managing safer sex depends upon personal goal setting and the exercise of interactional micro-skills to intervene in and direct sexual encounters. Thus, effective sex education should highlight the social realities of romantic and sexual relationships, focus on the existence of choices, acknowledge goal conflict, and highlight the impact of social context on risk taking, while also promoting the development of relevant social skills.

2.3 Changing cognitions and nurturing relevant interactive skills

A variety of social cognition and self-regulation models have outlined psychological antecedents of action that can be viewed as targets for change by health educators (see Conner and Norman 1996 for overviews; Abraham *et al.* 1998a). These models have been applied to safer sexual behaviour, including condom use, and have been found to be useful predictors (for example Fisher *et al.* 1995; Godin and Kok 1996; Sheeran *et al.* 1999).

Applications of these models suggest that preventive action is most likely when people hold a series of specific beliefs about recommended action. These include acceptance that they, and people like them, are susceptible to a preventable risk (Janz and Becker 1984) and that recommended prevention action is effective and will have more positive than negative consequences (Fishbein and Ajzen 1975). Feeling confident that one can overcome barriers to undertaking the action by, for example, recognizing likely impediments and developing skills and plans to overcome them, is also important (Bandura 1986; Ajzen 1991; Bandura 1997, 1998). In addition, the perception that others are acting in a similar manner and approve of the recommended action, especially those whose approval is valued, is likely to prompt intention formation and action (Fishbein and Ajzen 1975; Boyd and Wandersman 1991). Such beliefs prompt intentions to take recommended action. Enactment of such intentions is more likely when people make specific plans about when and where they will initiate action (Gollwitzer 1993; Gollwitzer and Oettingen 1998) and when they anticipate feelings of regret if they do not act (Richard *et al.* 1996).

Such research suggests that sex education should highlight the risks of pregnancy, STIs, emotional upset and regret, and should recommend delaying sexual intercourse until both partners feel psychologically ready. Programmes should also emphasize positive aspects of condom and contraceptive use, including their effectiveness in preventing STIs and pregnancy. At the same time, the difficulties young people face in acquiring, carrying, negotiating and using condoms and other contraceptives need to be acknowledged, and practical ways of overcoming them rehearsed. The approval of condom and contraceptive use by potential sexual partners should also be emphasized, by presenting findings that suggest widespread approval among young people (for example Abraham *et al.* 1992).

Feeling confident that one can perform an action successfully is fundamental to the formation and enactment of intentions (Ajzen 1998; Bandura 1998). Bandura (1997) identifies a number of sources of self-efficacy. The first is personal mastery experiences – for example, practising opening and handling condoms in class, and successfully discussing sexual risks with members of the opposite sex. Second, people may develop feelings of self-efficacy through observing others' successful actions – for example, a video of people negotiating what they want in a romantic or sexual encounter (whether refusing sexual advances or ensuring condom use). Such observation has been found to be especially powerful if observers perceive the model to be similar to themselves in ability, attitudes or group membership – for example, a person of their own age, sex, cultural grouping and nationality.

Finally, people may be persuaded of their abilities – for example, by reflecting on past successes and receiving positive feedback about present performances. Thus, exercises that encourage recognition of problem-solving abilities in relation to romantic and sexual encounters and involve cooperative consideration of sexual issues with members of the opposite sex are likely to build confidence.

Translating intentions into action is facilitated by the development of detailed and realistic plans (Gollwitzer 1993; Miller *et al.* 1993). Consequently, an important aspect of enhancing self-efficacy will be a realistic appraisal of how relevant social situations unfold (for example, who is likely to say what, when) and of what opportunities exist for taking and losing control (for example, insisting on what you want and listening to others). By rehearsing and planning, young people can be better prepared to interrupt potentially difficult scripts through becoming sensitized to key situational and social cues, including non-verbal behaviour. 'Trigger video' scenarios, in which scenes unfold gradually and can be discussed and evaluated at particular stages, can prompt such rehearsal. Scenes of this sort are included in the SHARE pack in the form of the *Knowing the Score* video,[1] and are designed to help people consider how decisions and actions in romantic and sexual interaction can result in different outcomes. The procedure involves observation of peers acting competently and effectively, and highlights social settings in which specific actions need to be taken. The scenarios include young women refusing sex and insisting on using condoms, as well as joint planning of safer sex. Pilot work assessing the exercises suggested that they worked well, sometimes prompting absorbing discussion that had to be curtailed by teachers.

Rehearsal is especially important for those inexperienced in managing romantic and sexual relationships because both partners may strive to maintain ambiguity about their intentions at first (Kent *et al.* 1990). The desire to become sexually involved is often concealed, so that rejection and humiliation are minimized if the wish is not mutual. Concealing sexual desire may maintain partner approval and also legitimize negotiation of romantic discourses involving being 'carried away'. Little wonder that first sexual intercourse is often unplanned (Johnson *et al.* 1994) and contraception is often discussed only afterwards (Wight 1993a). Negotiating ambiguity delays discussion of sexual risks and postpones consideration of condom use until sexual activity is initiated when, if a condom is not available, it may be difficult to negotiate pausing in order to acquire one. Conversely, if one partner is explicit about their wish to have sex, discussion of the desirability of sex and appropriate precautions becomes legitimate. Such explicit negotiation can allow better assessment of a partner's views and can establish a cooperative approach to negotiating a romantic relationship without sexual intercourse, or safer sex. Negotiations of this kind are modelled in the *Knowing the Score* video.

3 The intervention

Developing a research-based behaviour-change intervention does not guar-antee its acceptance by health educators or, in this case, schools. The pro-cesses involved in integrating a new programme into current provision are distinct from those involved in the development of materials. Yet unless the former are considered during development, the programme may never be widely, or faithfully, implemented, even if it is shown in trials to be effective. There is, however, relatively little research into how the manage-ment of programme acceptance and diffusion should influence programme development. Orlandi *et al.* (1990) argued that the diffusion of interven-tions should involve a collaborative partnership between the group pro-moting a programme and its potential users, operating through what they called a 'linkage system'. Schaalma *et al.* (1996) emphasized the importance of cooperation between researchers, school advisers and teachers in the development of school programmes, and underlined the need to pre-test materials in classroom settings. More recently, Bartholomew *et al.* (1998) have outlined a useful five-step framework for intervention development which considers implementation issues.

The SHARE team were conscious from the outset that the implications of research findings could challenge current educational practice and that programme costs and demands on curriculum time could threaten the sustainability and replicability of the programme. A teacher-led programme that conflicts with teachers' professional philosophy is unlikely to be adopted nationally, and costly interventions (such as involving outside professionals or organizing visits to local sexual health services) are likely to be dropped in the face of competing organizational demands. Potential conflicts meant that we had to give higher priority to some of our design principles than others and had to adapt our research-based materials to the constraints of the classroom (Wight and Abraham 2000).

3.1 Integrating research recommendations with current practice

Current health education practice is often designed 'to ensure that indi-viduals are able to exercise informed choice' (Department of Health 1992) and health education policy has focused on the interrelated goals of em-powering participants and raising their self-esteem (French and Adams 1986; Tones 1992). In school contexts this may promote educational pro-grammes in which teachers encourage students to set their own educational agendas (for example French 1990; Sex Education Forum 1997). These approaches conflict with research-based recommendations for standardized behaviour-specific advice. For example, Kirby *et al.* (1994: 355) observed that sex education programmes that 'emphasised clear behavioural values and norms' were more likely to be effective than those in which students are encouraged to draw their own conclusions. Research-based programmes should start with local needs assessments (Fisher and Fisher 1992; Bartholomew *et al.* 1998); research of this sort was conducted with Scottish teenagers before the SHARE programme was designed (Abraham *et al.* 1992; Wight 1993b; Wight and Scott 1994). However, class-specific sessions cannot be accommodated within standardized behaviour change programmes. Moreover, our own observations suggest that, in practice, it is difficult to negotiate sexual learning needs with teenage students in classroom settings (Wight 1999). Thus, the SHARE programme offers clear advice to teenagers: delay sexual intercourse until you are sure you (and your partner) are ready, and always use a condom until you plan to have children. The pack provides for optional extension exercises but schools are contracted to deliver the programme without modification. Thus, our first principle (concerning the application of research findings) and our third and fourth principles (regarding standardization and replicability) meant that the SHARE programme did not always conform to current practice.

We had to ensure that the programme was acceptable to the teachers who would deliver it. An important decision was the inclusion in the development team of a highly regarded sex education consultant who not only subscribed to an 'empowerment' approach to sex education (Dixon 1993) but also subscribed to the aims of the SHARE researchers. Hilary Dixon, the first author of the SHARE programme pack, played a key role as what Orlandi *et al.* (1990) call a 'linkage agent'. Her involvement boosted the credibility of the programme with both teachers and education officials and ensured that the teacher training course and session plans were fully adapted to the constraints of classroom management. The consultant also led the teacher training programme, which was designed to raise teachers' self-efficacy. Feedback suggests that the course was effective: 86 per cent of teachers judged it a very positive experience and a few commented that it was the best in-service training they had received.

3.2 Overcoming practical problems 1: the gendered construction of sexuality and classroom dynamics

A number of practical problems arose during the development of the pack and video, requiring adaptation of the SHARE programme (Wight and Abraham 2000). For example, encouraging a heterosocial perspective on sexuality in classroom settings proved somewhat more difficult than had been anticipated. A key objective of the programme was to improve young people's understanding of the attitudes and experiences of the opposite sex. The programme was initially designed to facilitate the process by moving from single-sex to mixed-sex discussion groups during sessions. This was strongly supported by students questioned in preliminary needs assessment research (Wight and Scott 1994) but proved problematic during piloting.

Feedback discussions revealed two main reasons for the failure. First, the very norms that some of the exercises aimed to reveal dominated classroom discussion and prevented reflexive insight into their operation. In all-male group discussions few boys felt sufficiently secure to go beyond conventional expressions of masculinity and seriously explore their masculine identities, despite agreeing ground rules at the start of the course. For example, in a feedback discussion two boys noted:

> B1: I mean if you do talk about what you feel like, say if you're talking about caring and loving and stuff like that, and then you go away with your pals, a few of them, not all of them, will just go 'What was that crap you were talking about?' It's the macho image.
> B2: Nothing any guy says to another guy is true. They're all making it up.

The single-sex groups were lively, however, compared with the whole class plenaries and the mixed-sex groups that followed, which were often painfully quiet. The operation of masculine norms was also evident, with boys censoring their views before sharing them with girls or the teacher, knowing that they would otherwise be perceived as sexist and offensive. For instance, when boys in one group were asked to feed back their answers from a work sheet concerning attractiveness, they read 'Boys like girls with nice personalities' instead of what they had written: 'Boys like girls with big tits'. This example also illustrates young people's difficulties in finding socially acceptable vocabulary to discuss sexual desire in classroom settings.

The classroom itself is a highly salient social context for students, and their relationships with classmates and teachers regulate their participation in any educational programme. Feedback revealed how aware students were of the operation of these normative influences on their behaviour, including self and group censorship. For example, boys could reflect on how they presented themselves differently according to whether they were with other boys, with girls in class, or alone with their girlfriends. They noted, for example, that:

> B3: You're mair [more] Jack the Lad kind of thing [in the class], ken [you know]. You'd speak, like, just yourself with your bird.

and

> B4: You'd show respect to your girlfriend, ken, or you'd get a slap in the chops . . . Not that you wouldnae respect the lassies in the class but . . . You'd open out more to girlfriends than to the class.

In the revised SHARE pack the first four sessions employed single-sex groups but after session four classes were divided into mixed groups to which students were allocated by the teacher (to avoid speculation about self-chosen membership indicating romantic involvement or sexual attraction). Our feedback data supported the use of mixed-sex groups, suggesting that:

- boys worked better in small mixed groups (typically two girls, two boys) because they were liberated from defensive masculine norms, which dominated discourse in the all-male groups, allowing them to question the predominant norms of gendered sexuality
- boys also worked better in mixed groups because, in general, girls were more willing to apply themselves to the programme exercises
- participants sometimes became involved and interested in opposite gender perspectives through discussing issues with the opposite sex.

Questionnaire data revealed that three-quarters of both girls and boys liked working in these mixed groups. Girls observed that:

> It was good. Sometimes it was really funny. The boys opened up a little and you found that some of them had a sensitive side to their personality.

and

> I think that this was a great idea! You learn more about the type of people boys are and how they feel. It's better than getting just one sex's view.

Moreover, half the respondents reported that they now felt more confident to talk about sex with the opposite sex than they had done before the course.

> The course has made me more confident about talking about sex. I honestly think I could talk to the opposite sex about sex now. I don't think I would have been able to before the course, though.

This is important because, as we noted above, communication between partners about STI risk and condom use is a powerful predictor of contraceptive and STI protection (for example Sheeran *et al.* 1999). Therefore, to the extent that the programme can engender mixed-sex discourses and enhance self-efficacy in relation to discussion of sexual matters, it is laying the foundations for the social skills necessary to ensure safer sex in the future.

3.3 Overcoming practical problems 2: skill development work in classrooms

SHARE also sought to introduce students to condom acquisition and use. Exercises were designed to encourage positive attitudes towards carrying and use, to reduce anticipated embarrassment in relation to acquisition, and to enhance self-efficacy in relation to acquiring and handling condoms. Initial discussions with educational managers were discouraging, suggesting that condom-related exercises would be unacceptable in many Scottish schools (Wight and Scott 1994). However, piloting revealed that the session on learning how to use condoms correctly worked well in classrooms and received much praise from teachers. This was confirmed in both pilots. Moreover, during recruitment for the randomized controlled trial, 48 schools were approached and neither the 25 that participated nor those that declined mentioned the condom-handling exercises in their considerations about whether to take part.

We attribute the acceptability of the condom-handling session to the credibility of the SHARE team and to the success of the teacher training course, which gave teachers confidence to deliver the exercises without fear of embarrassment or pupil disruption. However, despite being able to demonstrate correct condom use in the classroom, homework exercises involving acquisition of condoms were found to be unacceptable. This was unfortunate. Providing young people with an excuse to buy, borrow or pick up condoms that minimizes personal embarrassment (that is, 'I had to do it for my homework') is a useful way to encourage practice of these skills. Barriers to acquisition and carrying are likely to be reduced in the future once a young person has tried and succeeded. Instead of homework, SHARE relies on informing students where they can acquire condoms and on observational learning through video sequences depicting young people collecting condoms at a clinic, carrying them and borrowing them from their friends.

As we have noted, condom acquisition and handling skills must be deployed in the context of social skills that enable young people to discuss condom and contraceptive use. In order to facilitate development of these skills, SHARE initially incorporated a series of progressively demanding role-play exercises designed both to sensitize students to the dynamics of unfolding social scripts in potentially sexual encounters and to practise responses that would allow them to make personal decisions. For example, in the second year, one session focused on anticipating sexual risk-taking from situational cues while another addressed the issue of power in heterosexual relationships. These sessions sought to develop planning and resistance skills as well as to establish the unacceptability of exerting sexual pressure.

The first pilot revealed that role-play exercises rarely worked well. Students found it difficult to think of useful lines, or, more often, did not take the exercise seriously and disrupted it or refused to take part. Teachers found it extremely difficult to rectify these problems, even though they had practised the exercises during teacher training. Several factors contributed to this problem. First, students lacked sexual experience. This meant that many failed to appreciate that the explicit negotiation of personal agendas or condom use might be difficult in romantic/sexual encounters. Consequently, they did not understand the need for rehearsal and found improvisation of sexual negotiation challenging. Second, despite efforts to distance students from their characters, concerns about the interpersonal consequences of having one's words and actions attributed to oneself rather than one's character inhibited adoption of scripted roles with classmates under peer surveillance. Third, role play may involve unwanted self-disclosure. Students may be rightly concerned that character improvisation may betray the limits or depth of their own experience. Thus, overall, limited sexual experience and the classroom context rendered role play difficult and socially threatening.

The solution to this problem is not obvious. If role plays are desexualized then they no longer provide the required skill-development opportunities, may be boring, and may appear out of place in sex education sessions. Rote learning of responses is also unlikely to work. For example, in an attempt to reduce personal involvement in the role-play sessions, we introduced much more structured exercises. Some were based on Barth's *Reducing the Risk* (Barth 1989), which had been evaluated as effective in the USA (Kirby *et al.* 1991). In Scottish schools, however, the repetition of lines was treated with derision, even by cooperative classes, and the exercises had to be abandoned. This may reflect cultural differences in students' expectations of teaching methods.

The SHARE approach to this problem was (as we have noted) to rely on observation of interaction sequences on video, to stop them, and to discuss how well the characters handled the situations and what they should have said and done differently. This is less personally involving than role-playing interactive sequences, but the cognitive rehearsal of negotiation and situation management should, nevertheless, prompt planning, provide ready-made templates for asserting control, and sensitize students to potentially upsetting interactions. This approach has not, however, entirely resolved problems associated with developing such social skills in classrooms. Despite the success of the training course, continuing evaluation has revealed that teachers feel least confident about delivering this part of the programme. Resistance from students is still evident, some preferring to watch video sequences passively rather than discuss characters' feelings and actions. This undermines the effectiveness of the sessions and challenges teachers' self-efficacy. There is also evidence that students, and some teachers, remain to be convinced of the need to develop sex-specific negotiation and refusal skills in school. Thus, further work will be required if the development of action planning and negotiation skills relevant to the management of romantic and sexual relationships is to be integrated fully into sex education in Scottish schools. Yet the development of such skills is likely to be a prerequisite to promoting delayed sexual intercourse and the proper use of condoms and contraception. We recommend that the role of schools in developing such skills is considered further by those involved in planning the provision of sex education and in formulating public health policy.

4 Discussion: implications for theory, policy and practice

The process of developing the SHARE programme followed four design principles. This resulted in a theoretically informed programme, but one that was tempered by teachers' concerns and the practical constraints of classroom management. The programme applies insights from social cognition models and other theoretical frameworks in the social sciences. Many excellent existing sex education materials were incorporated, but research findings and the requirement to standardize delivery in order to facilitate rigorous evaluation meant that the programme diverged from some commonly accepted principles of sex education. In particular, it focused on behaviour-specific issues and skills, rather than raising general self-esteem, and offered clear advice rather than empowering students to draw their own conclusions. The resulting programme is research-based, practical and sustainable within present educational budgets. Whether it is more effective than existing provision will be determined by a randomized controlled trial due to report in the near future. Whatever the outcome of that evaluation, the development and implementation of the SHARE programme has highlighted the need for a clearer consensus on the role of schools in developing the skills required to manage romantic and sexual encounters successfully. Research can highlight the skills required but the question of how a society encourages the development of those skills among teenagers remains a social, political and ethical question.

Acknowledgements

The authors would like to thank the Health Education Board for Scotland, which funded the development of SHARE and the Medical Research Council, which is funding the randomized controlled trial.

Note

1 *Knowing the Score: The SHARE Video* was produced and directed by Charles Abraham and Sandy Reid. It employs a scenario-based, stop-and-discuss format involving teenage actors and was inspired by the successful Dutch *Long Live Love* video package (Schaalma *et al.* 1996).

References

Abraham, C. and Sheeran, P. (1994) Modelling and modifying young heterosexuals' HIV-preventive behaviour: a review of theories, findings and educational implications, *Patient Education and Counselling*, 23: 173–86.

Abraham, C. and Wight, D. (1996) Developing HIV-preventive behavioural interventions for young people in Scotland, *International Journal of STD and AIDS*, 7(Supplement 2): 39–42.

Abraham, C., Sheeran, P. and Johnston, M. (1998a) From health beliefs to self-regulation: theoretical advances in the psychology of action control, *Psychology and Health*, 13: 569–91.

Abraham, C., Sheeran, P. and Orbell, S. (1998b) Can social cognitive models contribute to the effectiveness of HIV-preventive behavioural interventions? A brief review of the literature and a reply to Joffe (1996; 1997) and Fife-Shaw (1997), *British Journal of Medical Psychology*, 71: 297–310.

Abraham, C., Sheeran, P., Spears, R. and Abrams, D. (1992) Health beliefs and promotion of HIV-preventive intentions among teenagers: a Scottish perspective, *Health Psychology*, 11(6): 363–70.

Ajzen, I. (1991) The Theory of Planned Behavior, *Organizational Behavior and Human Decision Processes*, 50: 179–211.

Ajzen, I. (1998) Models of human social behavior and their application to health psychology, *Psychology and Health*, 13(4): 735–9.

Bandura, A. (1986) *Social Foundations of Thought and Action: A Social Cognitive Theory*. Englewood Cliffs, NJ: Prentice-Hall.

Bandura, A. (1997) *Self-Efficacy: The Exercise of Control*. New York: Freeman.

Bandura, A. (1998) Health promotion from the perspective of social cognitive theory, *Psychology and Health*, 13: 623–49.

Barth, R.P. (1989) *Reducing the Risk: Building Skills to Prevent Pregnancy*. Santa Cruz, CA: ETR.

Bartholomew, L.K., Parcel, G.S. and Kok, G. (1998) Intervention mapping: a process for developing theory- and evidence-based health education programs, *Health Education and Behavior*, 25: 545–63.

Berger, P. and Luckmann, T. (1966) *The Social Construction of Reality*. New York: Anchor.

Berridge, V. and Strong, P. (1993) *Aids and Contemporary History*. Cambridge: Cambridge University Press.

Biglan, A., Noell, J., Ochs, L., Smolkowski, K. and Metzle, C. (1995) Does sexual coercion play a role in the high-risk sexual behavior of adolescent and young adult women?, *Journal of Behavioral Medicine*, 18: 549–68.

Bloor, M., Barnard, M., Finlay, A. and McKeganey, N. (1993) HIV-related risk practices among Glasgow male prostitutes, *Medical Anthropology Quarterly*, 7: 1–19.

Boyd, B. and Wandersman, A. (1991) Predicting undergraduate condom use with the Fishbein and Ajzen and the Triandis Attitude-Behaviour models: implications for public health interventions, *Journal of Applied Social Psychology*, 21(22): 1810–30.

Bryan, A.D., Aiken, L.S. and West, S.G. (1996) Increasing condom use: evaluation of a theory-based intervention to prevent sexually transmitted diseases in young women, *Health Psychology*, 15: 371–82.

Bury, J. (1984) *Teenage Pregnancy in Britain*. London: Birth Control Trust.

Catania, J.A., Kegeles, S.M. and Coates, T.J. (1990) Towards an understanding of risk behaviour: an AIDS Risk Reduction Model (ARRM), *Health Education Quarterly*, 17: 53–72.

Christopher, F.S. and Roosa, M.W. (1991) An evaluation of an adolescent pregnancy prevention program: is 'Just say no' enough?, *Family Relations*, 39: 68–72.

Coggans, N., Shewan, D., Henderson, M. and Davies, J.B. (1991) *National Evaluation of Drug Education in Scotland*, Research Monograph 4. London: Institute for the Study of Drug Dependence.

Conner, M. and Norman, P. (eds) (1996) *Predicting Health Behaviour: Research and Practice with Social Cognition Models*. Buckingham: Open University Press.

Department of Health (1992) *The Health of the Nation: A Strategy for Health in England*. London: HMSO.

Dixon, H. (1993) *Yes, AIDS Again: A Handbook for Teachers*. Cambridge: Learning Development Aids.

Fishbein, M. and Ajzen, I. (1975) *Belief, Attitude, Intention and Behavior: An Introduction to Theory and Research*. Reading, MA: Addison-Wesley.

Fisher, B.J., Fisher, J.D. and Rye, B.J. (1995) Understanding and promoting AIDS-preventive behaviour: insights from the Theory of Reasoned Action, *Health Psychology*, 14(3): 255–64.

Fisher, J.D. and Fisher, W.A. (1992) Changing AIDS-risk behaviour, *Psychological Bulletin*, 111(3): 455–74.

French, J. (1990) Boundaries and horizons, the role of health education within health promotion, *Health Education Journal*, 49: 7–10.

French, J. and Adams, L. (1986) From analysis to synthesis, *Health Education Journal*, 45: 71–4.

Gagnon, J.H. and Simon, W. (1974) *Sexual Conduct: The Social Sources of Human Sexuality*. London: Hutchinson.

Godin, G. and Kok, G. (1996) The Theory of Planned Behavior: a review of its applications to health-related behaviors, *American Journal of Health Promotion*, 11(2): 87–98.

Gold, D. and Berger, C. (1983) The influence of psychological and situational factors on the contraceptive behaviour of single men: a review of the literature, *Population and Environment*, 6: 113–29.

Gollwitzer, P.M. (1993) Goal achievement: the role of intentions, in W. Stroebe and M. Hewstone (eds) *European Review of Social Psychology*, 4. Chichester: Wiley.

Gollwitzer, P.M. and Oettingen, G. (1998) The emergence and implementation of health goals, *Psychology and Health*, 13(4): 687–715.

Hawkes, G. (1996) *A Sociology of Society and Sexuality*. Buckingham: Open University Press.

Health Education Authority (1994) *Health Update 4: HIV/AIDS and Sexual Health*. London: Health Education Authority.

Holland, J., Ramazanoglu, C., Scott, S. and Thomson, R. (1990) Sex, gender and power: young women's sexuality in the shadow of AIDS, *Sociology of Health and Illness*, 12(3): 336–50.

Holland, J., Ramazanoglu, C., Sharpe, S. and Thomson, R. (1998) *The Male in the Head: Young People, Heterosexuality and Power*. London: Tufnell Press.

Jackson, S. (1982) *Childhood and Sexuality*. Oxford: Blackwell.

Jackson, S. and Scott, S. (eds) (1996) *Feminism and Sexuality: A Reader*. Edinburgh: Edinburgh University Press.

Janz, N. and Becker, M.H. (1984) The health belief model: a decade later, *Health Education Quarterly*, 11: 1–47.

Jemmott, J.B., Jemmott, L.S. and Fong, G.T. (1992) Reductions in HIV risk-associated sexual behaviours among black male adolescents: effects of an AIDS prevention intervention, *American Journal of Public Health*, 82: 372–7.

Johnson, A.M., Wadsworth, J., Wellings, K. and Field, J. (1994) *Sexual Attitudes and Lifestyles*. Oxford: Blackwell Scientific.

Kalichman, S.C., Carey, M.P. and Johnson, B.T. (1996) Prevention of sexually transmitted HIV infection: a meta-analytic review of the behavioral outcome literature, *American Behavioral Medicine*, 18: 6–15.

Kashima, Y., Gallois, C. and McCamish, M. (1993) The theory of reasoned action and cooperative behaviour: it takes two to use a condom, *British Journal of Social Psychology*, 32: 227–39.

Kent, V., Davies, M., Deverell, K. and Gottesman, S. (1990) Social interaction routines involved in heterosexual encounters: prelude to first intercourse. Paper presented at the Fourth Conference on Social Aspects of AIDS, South Bank Polytechnic, London, 7 April.

Kirby, D., Barth, R., Leland, N. and Fetro, J. (1991) Reducing the risk: a new curriculum to prevent sexual risk-taking, *Family Planning Perspectives*, 23: 253–63.

Kirby, D., Short, L., Collins, J. *et al.* (1994) School-based programs to reduce sexual risk behaviours: a review of effectiveness, *Public Health Reports*, 109: 339–60.

Leventhal, H. (1970) Findings and theory in the study of fear communications, in L. Berkowitz (ed.) *Advances in Experimental Social Psychology*, 5. New York: Academic Press.

McRobbie, A. (1996) More! New sexualities in girls' and women's magazines, in J. Curran, D. Morley and V. Walkerdine (eds) *Cultural Studies and Communication*. London: Edward Arnold.

Martin, B. (1981) *A Sociology of Contemporary Cultural Change*. Oxford: Blackwell.

Mellanby, A.R., Phelps, F.A., Crichton, N.J. and Tripp, J.H. (1995) School sex education: an experimental programme with educational and medical benefit, *British Medical Journal*, 311: 414–17.

Miller, L.C., Bettencourt, B.A., DeBro, S.C. and Hoffman, V. (1993) Negotiating safer sex: interpersonal dynamics, in J.B. Pryor and G.D. Reeder (eds) *The Social Psychology of HIV Infection*. Hillsdale, NJ: Lawrence Erlbaum.

Morgan, D. and Scott, S. (1993) Bodies in a social landscape, in S. Scott and D. Morgan (eds) *Body Matters: Essays on the Sociology of the Body*. Lewes: Falmer Press.

National Health Service Centre for Reviews and Dissemination (1997) Preventing and reducing the adverse effects of unintended teenage pregnancies, *Effective Health Care*, 3: 1.

Oakley, A., Fullerton, D., Holland, J. *et al.* (1995) Sexual health education interventions for young people: a methodological review, *British Medical Journal*, 310: 158–62.

Orlandi, M., Landers, C., Weston, R. and Haley, N. (1990) Diffusion of health promotion innovations, in K. Glanz, F.M. Lewis and B. Rimer (eds) *Health Behavior and Health Education*, 2nd edn. San Francisco, CA: Jossey-Bass.

Polit-O'Hara, D. and Kahn, J. (1985) Communication and contraceptive practices in adolescent couples, *Adolescence*, 20: 33–42.

Richard, R., van der Pligt, J. and de Vries, N.K. (1996) Anticipated regret and time perspective: changing sexual risk-taking behavior, *Journal of Behavioral Decision Making*, 3: 263–77.

Ross, M.W., Rigby, K., Rosser, B.R., Anagnostou, P. and Brown, M. (1990) The effect of a national campaign on attitudes toward AIDS, *AIDS Care*, 2: 339–46.

Rotheram-Borus, M.J., Koopman, C., Haignere, C. and Davies, M. (1991) Reducing HIV sexual risk behaviours among runaway adolescents, *Journal of the American Medical Association*, 266: 1237–41.

Royal College of Obstetricians and Gynaecologists (1991) *Report of the RCOG Working Party on Unplanned Pregnancy*. London: RCOG.

Schaalma, H., Kok, G., Bosker, R. *et al.* (1996) Planned development and evaluation of AIDS/STD education for secondary-school students in the Netherlands: short-term effects, *Health Education Quarterly*, 23: 469–87.

Scott, S. and Freeman, R. (1995) Prevention as a problem of modernity: the example of HIV and AIDS, in J. Gabe (ed.) *Medicine, Health and Risk: Sociological Approaches*. Oxford: Blackwell.

Scottish Needs Assessment Programme (1994) *SNAP Report, Teenage Pregnancy in Scotland*. Glasgow: Scottish Forum for Public Health Medicine, Glasgow University.

Sex Education Forum (1997) *Forum Factsheet 11: Supporting the Needs of Boys and Young Men in Sex and Relationships Education*. London: National Children's Bureau.

Sheeran, P., Abraham, C. and Orbell, S. (1999) Psychosocial correlates of condom use: a meta-analysis, *Psychological Bulletin*, 125: 90–132.

Sherr, L. (1987) An evaluation of the UK government health education campaign on AIDS, *Psychology and Health*, 1: 61–72.

Social Exclusion Unit (1999) *Teenage Pregnancy*, Cm 4342. London: The Stationery Office.

Tones, K. (1992) Empowerment and the promotion of health, *Journal of the Institute of Health Education*, 30: 4.

Walter, H.J. and Vaughan, M.S. (1993) AIDS risk reduction among a multiethnic sample of urban high school students, *Journal of the American Medical Association*, 270: 725–30.

Wellings, K. (1996) *Young Women's Magazines and Teenage Sex: a Working Paper*. London: Department of Public Health and Policy, London School of Hygiene and Tropical Medicine.

Wight, D. (1993a) Constraint or cognition? Young men and safer heterosexual sex, in P. Aggleton, P. Davies and G. Hart (eds) *AIDS: Facing the Second Decade*. London: Falmer Press.

Wight, D. (1993b) A re-assessment of health education on HIV/AIDS for young heterosexuals, *Health Education Research: Theory and Practice*, 8: 473–83.

Wight, D. (1994) Boys' thoughts and talk about sex in a working class locality of Glasgow, *Sociological Review*, 42: 703–37.

Wight, D. (1999) Limits to empowerment-based sex education, *Health Education*, 99: 233–43.

Wight, D. and Abraham, C. (2000) From psycho-social theory to sustainable classroom practice: developing a research-based teacher-delivered sex education programme, *Health Education Research*, 15: 25–38.

Wight, D. and Scott, S. (1994) *Mandates and Constraints on Sex Education in the East of Scotland. Report to Health Education Board for Scotland.* London: Medical Research Council.

Wight, D. and Scott, S. (1996) *The Development and Piloting of SHARE, a Teacher-led Sex Education Programme for S3 and S4. Report to Health Education Board for Scotland.* London: Medical Research Council.

Wight, D., Abraham, C. and Scott, S. (1998) Towards a psycho-social theoretical framework for sexual health promotion, *Health Education Research: Theory and Practice*, 13: 317–30.

Wight, D., Henderson, M., Raab, G. *et al.* (2000) Extent of regretted sexual intercourse among young teenagers in Scotland: a cross-sectional survey, *British Medical Journal*, 320: 1243–4.

3   LYNN B. MYERS AND
SUSIE FROST

SMOKING AND SMOKING CESSATION: MODIFYING PERCEPTIONS OF RISK

It has been estimated that 450 million of the world's present population will be killed by smoking-related diseases in the next 50 years. The beneficial effects of giving up smoking are considerable. For example, 10 years after quitting, the risk of lung cancer falls to half that in smokers. There are two types of interventions to help people to give up smoking: motivational interventions and treatment interventions. The intervention described in this chapter was aimed at motivation, and investigated the possibility of changing smokers' beliefs about their risk of contracting smoking-related diseases.

When smokers are compared with other smokers they tend to state that they are less likely to contract smoking-related diseases (that is, they exhibit comparative optimism). The current intervention attempted to 'debias' comparative optimism by requiring smokers to imagine a scenario in which they contract a smoking-related disease. The debiasing intervention had opposing effects depending on the starting baseline. After completing the debiasing intervention, those who originally demonstrated comparative optimism no longer did so, but those who did *not* originally exhibit comparative optimism were comparatively optimistic. It is concluded that, if smokers are comparatively optimistic for smoking-related diseases, an intervention that engages them about the severe consequences of smoking may be successful in motivating them to quit.

1 Smoking and smoking cessation

1.1 Epidemiological facts and consequences

Some 3 million people die each year from smoking-related diseases, half of them before the age of 70 (Peto *et al.* 1994). It has been estimated that, in developed countries in 1990, tobacco was responsible for 24 per cent of all male deaths and 7 per cent of all female deaths. Recent figures have suggested that each cigarette smoked costs 11 minutes of life (Shaw *et al.* 2000). Even though smoking has been regarded as largely a male problem, it kills over half a million women a year world-wide, and the rate is increasing rapidly. In several developed countries, such as the USA and the UK, cigarette smoking is now the single most preventable cause of premature death in women, accounting for at least one-third of all deaths in women aged 35–69 (Peto *et al.* 1994). While there are no precise estimates for *undeveloped* countries, the prevalence figures suggest that smoking-related deaths will be numerous. Male smoking in many parts of the developing world now exceeds 50 per cent – 63 per cent in a recent study in China, for example (Yang *et al.* 1999). Overall mortality estimates based on current smoking patterns indicate that 450 million of the world's present population will be killed by tobacco in the next 50 years. These predictions will be substantially wrong only if there are major changes in global smoking patterns: reducing current smoking by 50 per cent would avoid 20–30 million premature deaths in the first quarter of the century and about 150 million in the second quarter (Peto and Lopez 2000).

Smoking is associated with a large number of both fatal and non-fatal diseases (see Wald and Hackshaw 1996). For example, a 40-year prospective study of smoking-related mortality among 34,000 male British doctors (Doll *et al.* 1994) found that a number of fatal diseases were positively correlated with smoking. Relative risk figures were presented as relative risk of current cigarette smokers compared with lifelong non-smokers. *Diseases where increased risk was largely or entirely caused by smoking* were cancer of the lung (relative risk 15.0), upper respiratory sites (relative risk 24.0), bladder (relative risk 2.3) and pancreas (relative risk 2.2); ischaemic heart disease (relative risk 1.6) and aortic aneurism (relative risk 4.1); and chronic obstructive lung disease (relative risk 12.7). *Increased risk partly caused by smoking* included cancer of the oesophagus (relative risk 7.5), stomach (relative risk 1.7) and kidney (relative risk 2.1); leukaemia (relative risk 1.8); stroke (relative risk 1.3) and pneumonia (relative risk 1.9). A study in the USA of more than 1 million men and women aged 35 and over found very similar evidence there (Surgeon General Report 1989).

A number of *non-fatal* diseases have also been shown to be associated with smoking. For example, peripheral vascular disease among 45–74-year-olds is almost entirely due to smoking (relative risk 2.0) (see Wald and

Hackshaw 1996 for a review), and there are also associations with disorders in pregnancy. These include spontaneous abortion (relative risk 1.28: Department of Health and Social Security 1988), ectopic pregnancy (relative risk 2.20: Campbell 1992) and congenital limb reduction defects (relative risk 2.10: Czeizel *et al.* 1994). Women who smoke during pregnancy also pass on harmful carcinogens to their baby (Hechr *et al.* 1998).

Although cigar smoking is seen as safer than cigarette smoking, it too is associated with increased risk of disease. For example, Iribaren *et al.* (1999) reported that cigar smokers were at higher risk of coronary heart disease (relative risk 1.27), chronic obstructive lung disease (relative risk 1.45) and cancers of the upper aerodigestive tract (relative risk 2.02) and lung (relative risk 2.14). Environmental tobacco smoke (or passive smoking) is also a potential health hazard. It has been estimated that a non-smoker living or working in a very smoky environment for a prolonged period is 20–30 per cent more likely to get lung cancer than a non-smoker who has not been persistently exposed to a smoky environment (Hackshaw *et al.* 1997) and 25 per cent more likely to suffer from coronary heart disease (He *et al.* 1999). In children, passive smoking is associated with a 25 per cent increase in the risk of chronic respiratory disease and a 50–100 per cent increase in the risk of acute respiratory illness (Law and Hackshaw 1996). Passive smoking in early pregnancy has been shown to double a woman's risk of delivering a small-for-gestational-age infant, independent of potential confounding factors such as age, height, weight and mother's smoking behaviour (Dejin-Karlsson *et al.* 1998).

Unsurprisingly, the cost of smoking is very high. In the UK, for example, it has been estimated that smoking costs the National Health Service up to £1.7 billion each year (Buck *et al.* 1997). Against the overall trend, however, there appear to be *negative* correlations between smoking and a small number of diseases. For example, cigarette smoking and nicotine may prevent or ameliorate Parkinson's disease (Gorrell *et al.* 1999) and possibly Alzheimer's disease in people over 65 years (Hebert *et al.* 1992). However, the benefits from the protective effects of smoking are minute when measured against the premature mortality that smoking causes (for reviews see Baron 1996; Wald and Hackshaw 1996).

1.2 Factors associated with smoking

The onset of smoking typically occurs during adolescence. According to Thomas *et al.* (1998), 82 per cent of smokers take up the habit as teenagers. In developed countries almost all smokers have begun by the age of 18 (Brooke *et al.* 1989). Environmental factors appear to be particularly important. In one study of monozygote and same-sex dizygote twins, for example, the findings suggested that smoking is influenced primarily by environmental factors rather than genetic factors (Han *et al.* 1999). Among them are social influences. Mother's smoking and friends' smoking, for example, predict smoking initiation in adolescents (Epstein *et al.* 1999). Moreover, parental smoking has been identified as a significant predictor of the transition from experimental smoking to regular use (Flay *et al.* 1998). Furthermore, first cigarettes are usually smoked with friends, and having a best friend who smokes is a strong predictor of whether a young person becomes a smoker (Charlton and Blair 1989). In a review of 27 prospective studies, onset was shown to be associated with socio-economic status, school bonding and peer bonding, peer smoking and approval, refusal skills, self-efficacy, intentions and self-esteem (Conrad *et al.* 1992). Tobacco is, of course, addictive, and within two or three years of starting to smoke, children report typical withdrawal symptoms when they try to give up (McNeill 1991).

In developed countries, smoking is associated with low income, low job status, unemployment, poor academic achievement and underprivileged background (for example Davis 1987; Montgomery *et al.* 1998; Pierce *et al.* 1998). As smokers die or quit, the tobacco industry has to recruit new young smokers to maintain its profits, especially in new markets such as developing countries and Eastern Europe (Amos 1996). Although the industry argues that cigarette advertisements do not encourage smoking but merely affect choice, research in developed countries shows that children can identify the brands in advertisements and that brand awareness is a strong predictor of future smoking (Aitkin 1988).

1.3 Previous interventions and why our own intervention was needed

The beneficial effects of giving up smoking are considerable: 24 hours after quitting, the smoker's lungs start to clear out mucus and debris; 2–12 weeks later, circulation improves throughout the body; and within 3–9 months, lung function increases by 5–10 per cent. In 5 years, the risk of suffering a myocardial infarction falls to half that in a smoker and in 10 years the risk is the same as in someone who has never smoked. Ten years after quitting, the risk of lung cancer falls to half that in smokers (QUIT 1996). In a recent paper, Peto *et al.* (2000) contrasted the results from two studies (1950 and 1990) of smoking cessation and lung cancer in the UK. They reported that people who quit smoking, even well into their middle age, avoid much of the risk of developing lung cancer, and if they stop before middle age the risk can be reduced to less than 10 per cent. For example, for men who quit smoking at ages 30, 40, 50 and 60, the cumulative risks of lung cancer by 75 years are 2 per cent, 3 per cent, 6 per cent and 10 per cent respectively.

Although seven out of ten adults say they would like to give up smoking (Freeth 1998), relapse rates are high. In countries such as the USA and UK, the rate of success in smoking cessation is typically 30 per cent (Shiffman 1993). Around 90 per cent of self-quitters relapse within three months, and the majority of early relapses are attributed to nicotine withdrawal syndrome, characterized by increased irritability, depression, anxiety, hunger, and inability to concentrate (Foulds 1999).

Over the past few decades, numerous interventions have been designed to encourage smokers to quit. As it is beyond the scope of the chapter to review them all, this section will focus on overall strategies. Strategies generally aim for two targets: motivation and treatment. Motivational interventions (for example media campaigns) are designed to encourage people to try to stop smoking, and treatment interventions (for example nicotine replacement) aim to increase the chances that an attempt to quit will be successful (see Foulds 1999 for a review). National policies generally try to influence both motivation and treatment (for example Department of Health 1998).

Motivational interventions
One method of motivating smokers to quit is through tobacco control. This includes legislation to ban tobacco advertising and sales to young people, health education, taxation to increase cigarette prices, restriction of smoking in public places, and product modification through the regulation of nicotine and tar content (see Reid 1996 for a review). California, for example, in 1989, introduced a package of motivational measures, including a mass media campaign. By 1993 tobacco consumption had fallen by half, and in 1996 the adult smoking rate was 18 per cent, compared to 22 per cent in the rest of the USA (Pierce *et al.* 1998). However, another large-scale community intervention in the USA, the Community Intervention Trial for Smoking Cessation (COMMIT), which took place over 4 years and involved 22 communities (half receiving a community intervention and half acting as controls), indicated no difference in the cessation rate for heavy smokers (COMMIT Research Group 1995a, 1995b). Foulds (1996) suggested that the results might have occurred because, in communities or countries where the health education message for anti-smoking is accepted and motivation for quitting is already high, motivational interventions will produce only small effects and will have a negligible impact on heavy, highly addicted smokers (see also Surgeon General Report 2000). In developed countries, the focus may need to be on individual treatment interventions, including specialist smoking clinics and strategies to improve self-quit attempts.

Treatment interventions
Studies have suggested that at least half of smokers who try to quit with the help of their family doctor experience withdrawal symptoms that meet the diagnostic criteria for nicotine withdrawal syndrome (for example Hughes 1992). Treatment interventions using Nicotine Replacement Therapy (NRT),

in the form of skin patch, gum, nasal spray and inhaler, have produced higher levels of abstinence than placebo interventions (Killen *et al.* 1997). In particular, transdermal nicotine patches have been associated with lower relapse rates (Killen *et al.* 1997) and fewer patient adherence problems and adverse effects (Mielke *et al.* 1997). Even when controlling for potential confounding variables, such as motivational support from health professionals, NRT doubles the probability of quitting (Raw *et al.* 1998).

Psychological interventions
Social cognition models and variables have been shown to be useful for both motivation and treatment interventions. For example, the Theory of Planned Behaviour (Ajzen 1985) has had some success in explaining smoking intentions and behaviour in adolescents (for example Maher and Rickwood 1997; O'Callaghan *et al.* 1999), in the general population (Godin *et al.* 1992) and in pregnant women (Godin *et al.* 1992). Self-efficacy has been shown to be a good predictor of smoking abstinence. For example, in a group cessation programme, post-treatment self-efficacy predicted abstinence at six months (Stuart *et al.* 1994) and was the strongest predictor ten months after a quit attempt (Kavanagh *et al.* 1993). Interventions based on the Transtheoretical Model (for example Prochaska *et al.* 1992) have had some success in adults (for example Velicer *et al.* 1999), but not in adolescents (Aveyard *et al.* 1999).

2 Theoretical perspective: risk perceptions and optimistic bias

Our own intervention was aimed at motivation, and investigated the possibility of changing smokers' beliefs about their risk of contracting smoking-related diseases. The central concept was 'unrealistic optimism', which Weinstein (1980) coined for the belief that negative events are *less* likely to happen to us than to others, while positive events are *more* likely to happen to us than to others. Unrealistic optimism is also known as 'optimistic bias' (Weinstein 1989) and has been reported for a multitude of events (see Hoorens 1994; Weinstein 1998b). *Health-related* events include the risk of skin cancer (for example Eiser and Arnold 1999), AIDS (for example Joseph *et al.* 1987), asthma (for example Peterson and De Avila 1995), heart attack (Weinstein 1982) and genetic risks (Welkenhuysen *et al.* 1997). The concept's importance in the present context is that inaccurate perceptions of risk and susceptibility may help to explain why people do not always practise healthy behaviours (Weinstein 1983, 1984).

While there is often an optimistic bias at the *group* level, *individuals* will exhibit varying degrees of optimism: some may be optimistic, some may be realistic, and some may be pessimistic (see for example Myers and Brewin

1996; Myers 1999). The intervention described in this chapter was an attempt to 'debias' smokers by targeting their *individual* optimism. When we investigate individuals' perceptions of risk in this way, and do not know their actual risk, the use of the terms 'optimistic bias' and 'unrealistic optimism' are not appropriate, and the term 'comparative optimism' should be used instead (Weinstein and Klein 1996). 'Comparative risk' and 'comparative optimism' will therefore be used when we describe the intervention in the next section.

Smokers' comparative risk judgements have been investigated in numerous studies (see Sutton 1999 for a recent review). In a number of them, when smokers were compared with other smokers for their perceived risk of contracting smoking-related diseases (for example lung cancer, heart disease), an optimistic bias was demonstrated in both adults and adolescents (Hansen and Malotte 1986; Lee 1989; Boney McCoy *et al.* 1992; McKenna *et al.* 1993; Segerstrom *et al.* 1993; Borland 1997; Williams and Clarke 1997). However, not all studies have found the same effect. For example, smokers showed no evidence of optimistic bias for lung cancer and heart disease in Sutton (submitted-a, submitted-b); and, although men showed optimistic bias for lung cancer and heart disease in Myers and McKenna (1998), women did not. Nevertheless, in a review, Weinstein (1998a) concluded that, although there were some inconsistencies, smokers in general do tend to minimize their personal health risks.

2.1 Methods for 'debiasing' comparative optimism

Research has suggested that perceptions of invulnerability, such as optimistic bias, are resistant to change (Weinstein *et al.* 1991; Weinstein and Klein 1994). However, there has been some success in 'debiasing' *comparative* risk judgements. For example, when drivers were told that they would be made *accountable* for their decisions, their optimistic bias for having an accident as a driver was reduced (McKenna and Myers 1997). Further studies indicated that it is possible to modify perceptions of invulnerability by requiring participants to imagine a relevant scenario with *severe* consequences for which the participants are to *blame* (McKenna and Myers 1995; McKenna and Myers in preparation).

There is strong evidence to suggest that imagination tasks might be a useful debiasing strategy. Studies have shown that instructions to imagine an event are sufficient to increase expectations of that event (Carroll 1978; Anderson 1983). In Anderson's study, the effect was found to persist for three days (Anderson 1983). It has also been shown that the ease of imagining the event affects the participant's belief in the likelihood of the event happening (Sherman *et al.* 1981; Gregory *et al.* 1985). Imagining self-relevant events can also influence participants' subsequent behaviours. When participants had to imagine working hard at a task and being either successful or unsuccessful, the group who imagined being successful performed the best in a subsequent task (Ruvolo and Markus 1992).

More recent studies, by McKenna and co-workers, have indicated that simply imagining an event is insufficient to debias perceptions of invulnerability (for example the likelihood of having a car accident as a driver). In a series of experiments on drivers' risk perceptions, the event (car accident) had to be severe, and the individual imagining the event (the driver) had to believe that they were to blame for the accident (for example McKenna 1994; McKenna and Myers in preparation), if successful debiasing was to take place. By involving the participants in this way, the debiasing effect on drivers has been shown to be present 24 hours after the debiasing intervention (McKenna and Myers 1995).

The intervention described in the following section attempted to extend the debiasing technique described above to smokers' perceptions of their health risks. Participants were asked to imagine a *severe* smoking-related disease happening to them, because of their smoking (that is, they were to *blame*), and to describe the consequences (McKenna and Myers 1996).

3 The intervention

Participating in the intervention were 43 adults (19 females and 24 males) aged between 18 and 44 years (mean = 22.33 years). They had smoked for between 1 and 28 years (mean = 5.97), and their consumption was between 1 and 30 cigarettes per day (mean = 12.05). In the first session, participants rated the likelihood of three events happening to them compared with the average smoker. These were developing lung cancer, having heart disease, and catching bronchitis. Ratings were on an 11-point scale, ranging from 1 anchored at 'Much less than average' to 11 anchored at 'Much more than average'. The midpoint (6) was labelled as 'Average'.

One to three months later, participants were invited back for the second part of the study, completing the debiasing questionnaire. Of the 88 people contacted, 43 responded. There were no significant differences between the responders and non-responders in years of smoking, number of cigarettes smoked per day, or initial ratings of comparative risk for lung cancer, heart disease and bronchitis. Participants were presented with a questionnaire that required them to describe an imaginary health problem. To aid imagination, they answered a series of questions concerning the details of the illness and its effect on their personal relationships and social and work life. Specific instructions were as follows:

> You are asked to describe an imaginary severe health problem which develops during the next few years due to your smoking, that is, you are to blame. Please describe the health problem and the consequences

for your personal, social and work life. Please make the description as realistic as you can, but do not describe a health problem that you have experienced.

Following completion of the questionnaire, participants were asked again to rate the likelihood of the three health events happening to them compared to the average smoker.

Preliminary results indicated that there were no significant differences between number of cigarettes smoked per day on the two occasions, nor were there significant effects of gender for any of the three health events. Cigarettes smoked and gender were therefore ignored in the main analyses. Means, standard deviations and one-sample t-tests are shown in Table 3.1.

Comparisons with responses about the hypothetical average person were carried out using one-sample t-tests, comparing participants with the mid-point of the scale (6). At Time 1, there was no comparative optimism for any of the three health behaviours: lung cancer, heart disease and bronchitis. These findings are similar to those in other studies (Myers and McKenna 1998; Sutton submitted-a, submitted-b). At Time 2 there was comparative optimism for lung cancer but not for heart disease or bronchitis (see Table 3.1).

Responses were next divided into two groups for each health event: those responses that were optimistic at Time 1; and those responses that were non-optimistic at Time 1. A series of MANOVAs were computed, for Group (optimistic against non-optimistic) by Time (Time 1 against Time 2). For each health event, there was a significant effect of Group, no significant effect of Time, and a significant Group by Time interaction.

To investigate these findings further, comparative risk estimates were compared against the mid-point (6), using one-sample t-tests at Time 1 and Time 2 and paired t-tests for Time 1 against Time 2 (see Table 3.1). At Time 1, for all three health events, the optimistic groups were significantly comparatively optimistic, whereas the non-optimistic groups were all significantly comparatively pessimistic (see Table 3.1). For *lung cancer*, the group that began by being comparatively optimistic was significantly less optimistic at Time 2 than at Time 1, and at Time 2 they did not differ significantly from the average. The group that initially was comparatively pessimistic was significantly less pessimistic at Time 2 than at Time 1, and at Time 2 they rated themselves significantly less likely to suffer from lung cancer than the average, that is, they were comparatively optimistic. For *heart disease*, the group that initially was comparatively optimistic was significantly less optimistic at Time 2 than at Time 1, and at Time 2 they rated themselves as significantly more likely to suffer from heart disease than the average, that is, they were comparatively pessimistic. The group that began by being comparatively pessimistic was significantly less pessimistic at Time 2 than at Time 1, and at Time 2 they did not differ significantly

Table 3.1 Mean self-ratings and standard deviation and one-sample t-tests for comparative risk estimates at Time 1 and Time 2 for all participants, initially optimistic, and initially non-optimistic participants

Health event	Means and (standard deviations) Time 1		Means and (standard deviations) Time 2		Paired t-tests	One-sample t-tests Time 1	One-sample t-tests Time 2
Lung cancer							
Overall	5.93	(1.98)	5.44	(1.37)	1.34	−0.23	−2.68*
Initially optimistic (n = 14)	3.62	(1.04)	5.77	(0.93)	−8.64***	−8.23***	−0.90
Initially non-optimistic (n = 29)	6.93	(1.34)	5.30	(1.51)	4.84***	3.82**	−2.54*
Heart disease							
Overall	5.86	(2.12)	6.35	(1.88)	−1.02	−0.43	1.08
Initially optimistic (n = 17)	3.88	(0.39)	7.12	(2.18)	−5.93***	−8.80***	2.12*
Initially non-optimistic (n = 26)	7.15	(1.59)	5.85	(1.95)	−3.05**	3.70**	−0.40
Bronchitis							
Overall	5.95	(2.12)	6.05	(1.93)	−0.18	−1.40	1.60
Initially optimistic (n = 16)	3.87	(1.26)	6.94	(1.08)	−5.41***	−6.76***	2.53*
Initially non-optimistic (n = 27)	7.19	(1.64)	5.52	(1.99)	3.45**	3.75***	−1.26

Notes: * p < 0.05   ** p < 0.001   *** p < 0.001

from the average. For *bronchitis*, the group that initially was comparatively optimistic was significantly less optimistic at Time 2 than at Time 1, and at Time 2 they rated themselves as significantly more likely to suffer from bronchitis than the average, that is, they were comparatively pessimistic. The group that began by being comparatively pessimistic was significantly less pessimistic at Time 2 than at Time 1, and at Time 2 they did not differ significantly from the average.

In summary, the intervention was successful for the comparatively optimistic groups. Individuals who were originally comparatively optimistic for lung cancer did not exhibit comparative optimism after the intervention, and for heart disease and bronchitis there was a significant comparative pessimistic bias at Time 2. Thus for those individuals, the debiasing strategy worked as predicted. However, for the group that initially was comparatively pessimistic, the intervention had a different effect. At Time 2, for lung cancer they shifted to comparative optimism. In other words, a group of individuals who had not shown an optimistic bias and were 'debiased' before the intervention did show an optimistic bias after the intervention. For both heart disease and bronchitis, the comparatively pessimistic groups lost their pessimism and were neither pessimistic nor optimistic at Time 2.

Why were these results the 'opposite' of what was expected? It may be hypothesized that the group who began as comparatively realistic/pessimistic and were aware of the personal risks of smoking found the intervention scenario (in which they had to imagine a severe smoking-related disease happening to them) so threatening that they reacted defensively, resulting in comparative optimism. Although high levels of comparative optimism have been reported in defensive individuals (Myers and Brewin 1996; Myers and Reynolds 2000), this explanation would have to be explored in future studies.

4 Discussion: implications for theory, policy and practice

Our results have important implications for media messages. If smokers are comparatively optimistic for smoking-related diseases, an intervention that engages them about the severe consequences of their behaviour may be successful in motivating them to quit. However, if smokers are realistic or pessimistic about their chances of contracting smoking-related diseases, such an intervention may have the opposite effect to the one intended. Therefore, in communities where the majority already tend to be motivated to quit, and are probably realistic or pessimistic about the chances of contracting smoking-related diseases, caution must be exercised in trying to change risk perception. It would be useful for future studies to identify communities where the majority of smokers are not motivated to quit and are comparatively optimistic about their chances of contracting smoking-related diseases.

It is likely that such communities may be found in developing countries and Eastern Europe where, at present, motivational interventions for quitting smoking are low. In such communities, media messages based on our debiasing technique may well be a useful tool.

Acknowledgements

We would like to thank Professor Stephen Sutton and Sarah Amponsah for help in the literature search. We would also like to thank Professor Frank McKenna for his dedication in enabling a successful debiasing technique to be developed.

References

Aitkin, P.P. (1988) *Children and Cigarette Advertising*, 8. Copenhagen: World Health Organization.
Ajzen, I. (1985) From intentions to actions: a theory of planned behaviour, in J. Kuhl and J. Beckman (eds) *Action Control: From Cognition to Behaviour*. Heidelberg: Springer.
Amos, A. (1996) Women and smoking, *British Medical Bulletin*, 52: 74–89.
Anderson, C.A. (1983) Imagination and expectation: the effect of imagining behavioral scripts on personal intentions, *Journal of Personality and Social Psychology*, 45: 293–305.
Aveyard, P., Cheng, K.K., Almond, J. *et al.* (1999) Cluster randomised control trial of expert system based on the transtheoretical model ('stages of change') model for smoking prevention and cessation in schools, *British Medical Journal*, 319: 948–53.
Baron, J.A. (1996) Beneficial effects of nicotine and cigarette smoking: the real, the possible and the spurious, *British Medical Bulletin*, 25: 58–73.
Boney McCoy, S., Gibbons, F.X., Reis, T.J. *et al.* (1992) Perceptions of smoking risk as a function of smoking status, *Journal of Behavioral Medicine*, 15: 469–88.
Borland, R. (1997) What do people's estimates of smoking related risk mean?, *Psychology and Health*, 12: 513–21.
Brooke, O.G., Anderson, H.R., Bland, J.M., Peacock, J.L. and Stewart, C. (1989) Effect on birth weight of smoking, alcohol, caffeine, socio-economic factors and psychosocial stress, *British Medical Journal*, 298: 795–801.
Buck, D., Godfrey, C., Parrott, S. and Raw, M. (1997) *Cost-effectiveness of Smoking Cessation Interventions*. London: Health Education Authority.
Campbell, O. (1992) Ectopic pregnancy and smoking: confounding or causality, in D. Poswillo and E. Alberman (eds) *Effects of Smoking on the Fetus, Neonate and Child*. Oxford: Oxford University Press.
Carroll, J.S. (1978) The effect of imagining an event on expectations for the event: an interpretation in terms of the availability heuristic, *Journal of Experimental Social Psychology*, 14: 88–96.

Charlton, A. and Blair, V. (1989) Predicting the onset of smoking in boys and girls, *Social Science and Medicine*, 29: 813–18.

COMMIT Research Group (1995a) Community Intervention Trial for Smoking Cessation (COMMIT): I. Cohort results from a four year community intervention, *American Journal of Public Health*, 85: 183–92.

COMMIT Research Group (1995b) Community Intervention Trial for Smoking Cessation (COMMIT): II. Cohort results from a four year community intervention, *American Journal of Public Health*, 85: 193–200.

Conrad, K.M., Flay, B.R. and Hill, D. (1992) Why children start smoking cigarettes: predictors of onset, *British Journal of Addiction*, 87: 1711–24.

Czeizel, A.E., Kojal, I. and Lenz, W. (1994) Smoking during pregnancy and congenital limb deficiency, *British Medical Journal*, 308: 1473–6.

Davis, R.M. (1987) Current trends in cigarette advertising and marketing, *New England Journal of Medicine*, 316: 725–32.

Dejin-Karlsson, E., Hanson, B.S., Oestergen, P., Sjoeberg, N. and Marsal, K. (1998) Does passive smoking in early pregnancy increase the risk of small-for-gestational age infants?, *American Journal of Public Health*, 88: 1523–7.

Department of Health (1998) *Smoking Kills: A White Paper on Tobacco*. London: Department of Health.

Department of Health and Social Security (1988) *Fourth Report of the Independent Scientific Committee on Smoking and Health*. London: HMSO.

Doll, R., Peto, R., Wheatley, K., Gray, R. and Sutherland, I. (1994) Mortality in relation to smoking: 40 years' observations on male British doctors, *British Medical Journal*, 309: 901–11.

Eiser, J.R. and Arnold, B.W.A. (1999) Out in the midday sun: risk behaviour and optimistic beliefs among residents and visitors on Tenerife, *Psychology and Health*, 14: 529–44.

Epstein, J.A., Botvin, G.J. and Diaz, T. (1999) Social influence and psychological determinants of smoking among inner-city adolescents, *Journal of Child and Adolescent Substance Abuse*, 8: 1–19.

Flay, B.R., Hu, F. and Richardson, J. (1998) Psychosocial predictors of different stages of cigarette smoking among high school students, *Preventive Medicine*, 27: 9–18.

Foulds, J. (1996) Strategies for smoking cessation, *British Medical Journal*, 52: 157–73.

Foulds, J. (1999) Nicotine Replacement Therapy: availability, abuse liability and dependence potential, in *Tackling Tobacco: Working Together for Better Health*. Cardiff: Health Promotion Wales.

Freeth, S. (1998) *Smoking-related Behaviour and Attitudes 1997: a Report on Records Using the ONS Omnibus Survey Produced on Behalf of the Department of Health*. London: The Stationery Office.

Godin, G., Valois, P., Lepage, L. and Desharnais, R. (1992) Predictors of smoking behaviour: an application of Ajzen's theory of planned behaviour, *British Journal of Addiction*, 87(9): 1335–43.

Gorrell, J.M., Rybicki, B.A., Johnson, C.C. and Peterson, E.L. (1999) Smoking and Parkinson's disease: a dose–response relationship, *Neurology*, 52: 115–19.

Gregory, W.L., Burroughs, W.J. and Ainslie, F.M. (1985) Self-relevant scenarios as an indirect means of attitude change, *Personality and Social Psychology Bulletin*, 11: 435–44.

Hackshaw, A.K., Law, M.R. and Wald, N.J. (1997) The accumulated evidence on lung cancer and environmental tobacco smoke, *British Medical Journal*, 315: 980–8.

Han, C., McGue, K. and Iacono, W.G. (1999) Lifetime tobacco, alcohol and other substance use in adolescent Minnesota twins: univariate and multivariate behavioral genetic analyses, *Addiction*, 94: 981–93.

Hansen, W.B. and Malotte, C.K. (1986) Perceived personal immunity: the development of beliefs about susceptibility and consequences of smoking, *Preventive Medicine*, 15: 363–72.

He, J., Vupputuri, S., Allen, K. *et al.* (1999) Passive smoking and the risk of coronary heart disease – a meta-analysis of epidemiologic studies, *New England Journal of Medicine*, 340: 920–6.

Hebert, L.E., Scherr, P.A., Beckett, L.A. *et al.* (1992) Relation of smoking and alcohol consumption to incidence of Alzheimer's Disease, *American Journal of Epidemiology*, 135: 347–55.

Hechr, S.S., Carmella, S.G., Chen, M.L. *et al.* (1998) Metabolites of the tobacco-specific lung carcinogen 4-(methylnitrosoamino)-1-(3-pyridyl)-1-butanone(nnk) in the urine of newborn infants, *Abstracts of Papers of the American Chemical Society*, 216: 32.

Hoorens, V. (1994) Unrealistic optimism in health and safety risks, in D.R. Rutter and L. Quine (eds) *Social Psychology and Health: European Perspectives*. Aldershot: Avebury.

Hughes, J.R. (1992) Tobacco withdrawal of self-quitters, *Journal of Consulting and Clinical Psychology*, 60: 331–4.

Iribaren, C., Tekawa, I.S., Sidney, S. and Friedman, G.D. (1999) Effect of cigar smoking on the risk of cardiovascular disease, chronic obstructive pulmonary disease and cancer in men, *New England Journal of Medicine*, 340: 1773–80.

Joseph, J.G., Montgomery, S.B., Emmons, C.-A. *et al.* (1987) Perceived risk of AIDS: assessing the behavioral and psychological consequences in a cohort of gay men, *Journal of Applied Social Psychology*, 17: 231–50.

Kavanagh, D.J., Pierce, J., Lo, S.K. and Shelley, L. (1993) Self-efficacy and social support as predictors of smoking after a quit attempt, *Psychology and Health*, 8(4): 231–42.

Killen, J.D., Fortmann, S.P., Davis, L. and Varady, A. (1997) Nicotine patch and self-help video for cigarette smoking cessation, *Journal of Consulting and Clinical Psychology*, 65: 663–72.

Law, M.R. and Hackshaw, A.K. (1996) Environmental tobacco smoke, *British Medical Bulletin*, 52: 22–34.

Lee, C. (1989) Perceptions of immunity to disease in adult smokers, *Journal of Behavioral Medicine*, 12: 267–77.

McKenna, F.P. (1994) Debiasing. Paper presented at the workshop on Optimism, Risk and Behavior, University of Amsterdam, July.

McKenna, F.P. and Myers, L.B. (1995) Changing risk perceptions: the role of the mass media, in G.B. Grayson (ed.) *Behavioural Research in Road Safety V*. Crowthorne: Transport Research Laboratory.

McKenna, F.P. and Myers, L.B. (1996) Smokers' perceptions of risk: can they be debiased?, *Proceedings of the British Psychological Society*, 4: 115.

McKenna, F.P. and Myers, L.B. (1997) Can accountability reduce or reverse existing illusory self assessments?, *British Journal of Psychology*, 88: 39–51.

McKenna, F.P. and Myers, L.B. (in preparation) Using imagination to debias drivers' risk perceptions.

McKenna, F.P., Warburton, D.M. and Winwood, M. (1993) Exploring the limits of optimism – the case of smokers' decision-making, *British Journal of Psychology*, 84: 389–94.

McNeill, A.D. (1991) The development of dependence on smoking in children, *British Journal of Addiction*, 86: 1041–54.

Maher, R.A. and Rickwood, D. (1997) The theory of planned behavior, domain specific self-efficacy and adolescent smoking, *Journal of Child and Adolescent Substance Abuse*, 6: 57–76.

Mielke, M.M., Jorenby, D.E. and Fiore, M.C. (1997) Achieving smoking cessation in nicotine-dependent individuals: practical guidelines, *CNS Drugs*, 8: 12–20.

Montgomery, S.M., Cook, D.G., Bartley, M.J. and Wadsworth, M.E.J. (1998) Unemployment, cigarette smoking, alcohol consumption and body weight in young British men, *European Journal of Public Health*, 8: 21–7.

Myers, L.B. (1999) Is optimistic bias for skin cancer realistic?, *Proceedings of the British Psychological Society*, 7: 25.

Myers, L.B. and Brewin, C.R. (1996) Illusions of well-being and the repressive coping style, *British Journal of Social Psychology*, 33: 443–57.

Myers, L.B. and McKenna, F.P. (1998) Gender differences in smokers' risk perception. Unpublished manuscript.

Myers, L.B. and Reynolds, R. (2000) How optimistic are repressors? The relationship between repressive coping, controllability, self-esteem and optimism for health-related events, *Psychology and Health*, 15: 667–88.

O'Callaghan, F.V., Callan, V.J. and Bagiolni, A. (1999) Cigarette use by adolescents: attitude behavior relationships, *Substance Use and Misuse*, 34: 455–68.

Peterson, C. and De Avila, M. (1995) Optimistic explanatory style and the perception of health problems, *Journal of Clinical Psychology*, 51: 128–32.

Peto, R. and Lopez, A.D. (2000) The future worldwide health effects of current smoking patterns, in C.E. Koop, C.E. Pearson and M.R. Schwartz (eds) *Critical Issues in Global Health*. New York: Jossey-Bass.

Peto, R., Lopez, A.D., Boreham, J., Thun, M. and Heath, C., Jr (1994) *Mortality from Smoking in Developed Countries: 1995–2000*. Oxford: Oxford University Press.

Peto, R., Darby, S., Deo, H. *et al.* (2000) Smoking, smoking cessation and lung cancer in the UK since 1950: combination of national statistics with two case control studies, *British Medical Journal*, 321: 323–9.

Pierce, J.P., Fiore, M.C., Novotny, T.E., Hatziandreu, E.J. and Davis, R.M. (1998) Trends in cigarette smoking in the United States: projections to the year 2000, *Journal of the American Medical Association*, 261: 61–5.

Prochaska, J.O., DiClemente, C.C. and Norcross, J.C. (1992) Measuring processes of how people change: applications to addictive behaviours, *American Psychologist*, 47: 1102–14.

QUIT (1996) *Helping Smokers to Quit*. London: QUIT.

Raw, M., McNeil, A. and West, R. (1998) Smoking cessation guidelines for health professionals: a guide to effective smoking cessation interventions for the health care system, *Thorax*, 53(Supplement 5).

Rcid, D. (1996) Tobacco control: overview, *British Medical Bulletin*, 52: 108–20.

Ruvolo, A.P. and Markus, H.R. (1992) Possible selves and performance – the power of self-relevant imagery, *Social Cognition*, 10: 95–124.

Segerstrom, S.C., McCarthy, W.J., Caskey, N.H., Gross, T.M. and Jarvik, M.E. (1993) Optimistic bias among cigarette smokers, *Journal of Applied Social Psychology*, 23(19): 1606–18.

Shaw, M., Mitchell, R. and Dorling, D. (2000) Time for a smoke? One cigarette reduces your life by 11 minutes, *British Medical Journal*, 320: 53.

Sherman, S.J., Skov, R.B., Hervitz, E.F. and Stock, C.B. (1981) The effects of explaining hypothetical future events: from possibility to actuality and beyond, *Journal of Experimental Social Psychology*, 17: 142–58.

Shiffman, S. (1993) Smoking cessation treatment; any progress?, *Journal of Clinical and Consulting Psychology*, 61: 718–22.

Stuart, K., Borland, R. and McMurray, N. (1994) Self-efficacy, health locus of control, and smoking cessation, *Addictive Behaviours*, 19: 1–12.

Surgeon General Report (1989) *Reducing the Health Consequences of Smoking: 25 Years of Progress*. Washington, DC: US Department of Health and Human Services.

Surgeon General Report (2000) *Treating Tobacco Use and Dependence: Summary*. Washington, DC: US Department of Health and Human Services.

Sutton, S.R. (1999) How accurate are smokers' perceptions of risk?, *Health, Risk and Society*, 1: 223–30.

Sutton, S.R. (submitted-a) Are smokers unrealistically optimistic about the health risks? Findings from two national surveys.

Sutton, S.R. (submitted-b) Influencing optimism in smokers by giving information about the average smoker.

Thomas, M., Walker, A., Wilmot, A. and Bennett, N. (1998) *Living in Britain: Results from the 1996 General Household Survey*. London: The Stationery Office.

Velicer, W.F., Prochaska, J.O., Fava, J.L., Laforge, R.G. and Rossi, J.S. (1999) Interactive versus noninteractive interventions and dose-response relationships for stage-matched smoking programs in a managed care setting, *Health Psychology*, 18(1): 21–8.

Wald, N.J. and Hackshaw, A.K. (1996) Cigarette smoking: an epidemiological overview, *British Medical Bulletin*, 52: 3–11.

Weinstein, N.D. (1980) Unrealistic optimism about future life events, *Journal of Personality and Social Psychology*, 39(5): 806–20.

Weinstein, N.D. (1982) Unrealistic optimism about susceptibility to health problems, *Journal of Behavioral Medicine*, 5(4): 441–60.

Weinstein, N.D. (1983) Reducing unrealistic optimism about illness susceptibility, *Health Psychology*, 2(1): 11–20.

Weinstein, N.D. (1984) Why it won't happen to me: perceptions of risk factors and susceptibility, *Health Psychology*, 3(5): 431–57.

Weinstein, N.D. (1989) Optimistic bias about personal risks, *Science*, 246: 1232–3.

Weinstein, N.D. (1998a) Accuracy of smokers' risk perceptions, *Annals of Behavioral Medicine*, 20: 135–40.

Weinstein, N.D. (1998b) References on optimistic biases about risk and future life events. Unpublished manuscript.

Weinstein, N.D. and Klein, W.M. (1994) Resistance of personal risk perceptions to debiasing manipulation, *Health Psychology*, 14: 132–40.

Weinstein, N.D. and Klein, W.M. (1996) Unrealistic optimism: present and future, *Journal of Social and Clinical Psychology*, 15(1): 1–8.

Weinstein, N.D., Sandman, P.M. and Roberts, N.E. (1991) Perceived susceptibility and self-protective behavior: a field experiment to encourage home radon testing, *Health Psychology*, 10: 25–33.

Welkenhuysen, M., Everskiebooms, G. and Dydewalle, G. (1997) Unrealistic optimism about specific genetic risks and perceived preventability, *Psychologica Belgica*, 37: 169–81.

Williams, T. and Clarke, V.A. (1997) Optimistic bias in beliefs about smoking, *Australian Journal of Psychology*, 49: 106–12.

Yang, G., Fan, L., Tan, J. *et al.* (1999) Smoking in China: findings of the 1996 National Prevalence Study, *Journal of the American Medical Association*, 282: 1247–53.

4 | NEIL D. WEINSTEIN AND
PETER M. SANDMAN

REDUCING THE RISKS OF EXPOSURE TO RADON GAS: AN APPLICATION OF THE PRECAUTION ADOPTION PROCESS MODEL

This chapter describes the Precaution Adoption Process Model (Weinstein and Sandman 1992), a framework for understanding situations in which people take deliberate actions to reduce health risks. In contrast to most theories of health behaviour, the PAPM describes the initiation of new behaviours in terms of progress through a sequence of qualitatively different stages. Stage theories differ in important respects from other theories used to explain health behaviours, and part of the goal of the chapter is to clarify these differences. To provide a concrete context for these discussions, most of the examples here will refer to the risk of lung cancer produced by exposure to radon gas.

1 Reducing the risks of exposure to radon gas

1.1 Radon as a controllable health hazard

Radon is an invisible, odourless, radioactive gas produced by the decay of small amounts of naturally occurring uranium in soil. It enters homes through foundation cracks and other openings. Radiation from the decay of radon can damage cells in the lungs, and radon is the second leading cause of lung cancer after smoking (US National Academy of Sciences 1988; US Environmental Protection Agency Office of Radiation Programs and US Department of Health and Human Services Centers for Disease Control 1992). Concentrations exceeding recommended action levels are present in about 6 per cent of homes in the United States (US Environmental Protection Agency

Office of Radiation Programs 1991, 1992) and high radon levels are found in many other countries.

Radon tests can be carried out by homeowners with a modest degree of effort. A single do-it-yourself test typically costs between $10 and $50. Testing is also provided by private companies. If elevated radon levels are found in a home, they can be reduced for a cost comparable to that of fixing a leaky roof or spraying for termites.

1.2 How traditional theories approach the issue of explaining and changing health behaviour

Since significant changes in behaviour seem to require conscious decision making, the theories used most frequently to explain individual preventive health behaviour (for example the Theory of Reasoned Action (Fishbein and Ajzen 1975; Ajzen and Fishbein 1980; Fishbein and Middlestadt 1989); the Theory of Planned Behaviour (Ajzen 1985; Ajzen and Madden 1986); the Health Belief Model (Rosenstock 1974; Janz and Becker 1984; Kirscht 1988); Protection Motivation Theory (Rogers 1983; Prentice-Dunn and Rogers 1986); Subjective Expected Utility Theory (Edwards 1954; Sutton 1982; Ronis 1992)) view action as the outcome of a cognitive process that weighs expected benefits against costs. The first main goal of these theories is to identify the variables – including beliefs, experiences, social pressures, and past behaviour – that have the greatest impact on such decisions.

The second goal of these theories is to predict behaviour. The theories combine the variables they have identified in an equation that is either prescribed by the theory or derived empirically from collected data (for examples see Weinstein 1993). Each theory has a single prediction equation. Substituting the variables into this equation leads to a single numerical value for each individual, and this value is interpreted as the relative probability that this person will act. Thus, the prediction rule places each person along a *continuum* of action likelihood, and such theories might be called 'continuum theories'. The goal of interventions, according to this perspective, is to move people along the continuum, increasing the probability of action, though action can occur from any point along the continuum. If different interventions increase the value of the prediction equation by the same amount, they are all expected to produce the same change in behaviour.

1.3 How stage theories approach the issue of explaining and changing behaviour

Many natural phenomena pass through qualitatively different stages, with different issues being important at each stage. Advocates of stage theories of health behaviour question whether change can be described by a single prediction equation. In effect, they suggest that we must try to understand a whole series of changes, identifying the relevant variables and the way in which they combine for each stage transition. Although this is much more complicated than finding a single prediction rule, it offers the possibility of greater effectiveness. An example may help make this claim clear.

Consider radon testing. A great many variables – social norms, knowledge, efficacy beliefs, risk perceptions – are likely to influence whether or not a person tests his or her home. However, given a list of such variables, how do we design a programme to encourage testing? Should every intervention address all relevant variables? Do certain topics (such as risk levels and vulnerability) need to be addressed before others (such as choosing and using radon test kits)? A stage theory of radon testing would specify an ordered set of categories into which people could be classified and identify the factors that could induce movement from one category to the next. Given such a theory, a health educator approaching a new population could identify the dominant stage or stages and focus available resources on those factors that are most important in moving people to the next stage. Thus, the greatest attraction of stage theories is the potential they offer for tailoring messages to audiences.

Continuum theories acknowledge quantitative differences among people in terms of their likelihood of action. The theories do not, however, acknowledge changes in the barriers that people must overcome to progress towards action. Certain variables are most important, and the goal of interventions is to maximize these variables for everyone. Thus, the notion of matching interventions to people is either incidental or completely missing in continuum theories.

Essential elements of stage theories

Stage theories of health behaviour have four principal elements (Weinstein *et al.* 1998b):

1 A category system to define the stages
   Stages are theoretical constructs. A 'prototype' can be defined for each stage, but we should remember that few people will match this ideal perfectly.
2 An ordering of the stages
   Stage theories assume that people must pass through all the stages to reach the end point of action or maintenance. However, progression is neither inevitable nor irreversible (cf. Bandura 1995).
3 Common barriers to change facing people in the same stage
   Stage ideas will be helpful in encouraging people to move towards action if people at one stage have to address similar issues before they can progress to the next stage.
4 Different barriers to change facing people in different stages
   If the factors producing movement towards action were the same regardless of a person's stage, the same intervention could be used for all, and the concept of stages would be superfluous.

The stages described by a theory are thought to apply to a wide range of behaviours. For example, the distinction between people who are undecided about acting and those who have decided to act may be important for all new health behaviours. Some of the barriers to progress between stages may also be common across health actions, but others may be action specific. Thus, the particular factors that help people decide to lose weight, may be quite different from the factors that help people decide to use condoms. A model that proposes a particular sequence of stages in the change process can be correct even if it has not identified the barriers at each stage. The stages constitute a framework that needs to be filled in by additional research.

How stage theories can be tested
A variety of approaches have been used to determine whether a particular behaviour change does pass through the sequence of stages described by a stage theory (Weinstein *et al.* 1998b). The most common approach, using cross-sectional data to look for differences between people thought to be in different stages, turns out to be a very poor test, since non-stage processes will also produce such differences. Comparing an intervention tailored to stage with a standard intervention is also a poor test, since tailoring usually involves personalization and extra attention. The latter ingredients, rather than the tailoring, could easily explain greater success in the tailored condition.

Much more definitive are experimental studies using matched and mismatched interventions. If it is true that different variables influence movement at different stages, treatments designed to influence these variables should be most effective when applied to people in the appropriate stage. Thus, individuals in a given stage should respond better to an intervention that is *matched* to their stage than to one that is *mismatched* (that is, matched to a different stage).

Only stage models predict that the sequencing of treatments is important. For maximum effectiveness, the sequence of interventions should follow the hypothesized sequence of stages. Consequently, sequence effects provide further evidence of a stage process. Unfortunately, because they require multiple interventions, they are quite difficult to implement and test.

An elegant data analysis method for testing whether different issues are significant at different stages has been developed by Hedeker *et al.* (1999). It can be used with experimental, prospective, and cross-sectional research designs.

2 Theoretical perspective: the Precaution Adoption Process Model

2.1 Description of the model

Several aspects of the theory were discussed in 1988 (Weinstein 1988), but the present formulation was first published in 1992 (Weinstein and Sandman

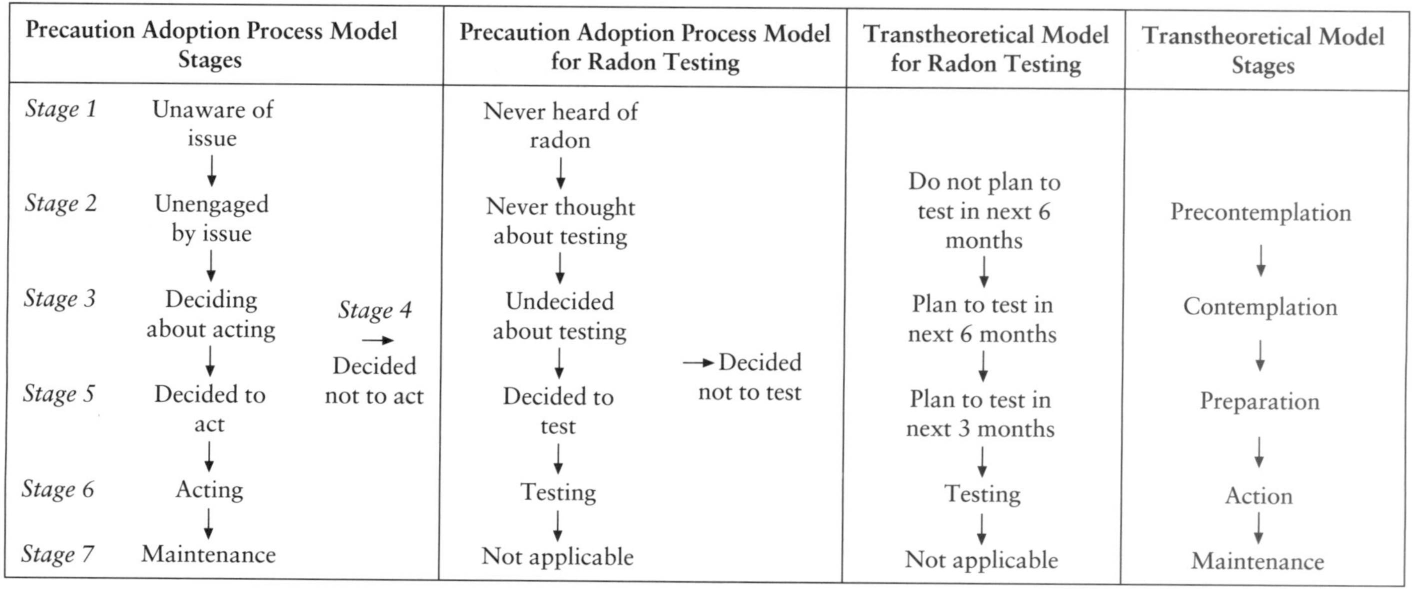

Precaution Adoption Process Model Stages		Precaution Adoption Process Model for Radon Testing	Transtheoretical Model for Radon Testing	Transtheoretical Model Stages
Stage 1	Unaware of issue	Never heard of radon		
	↓	↓		Precontemplation
				↓
Stage 2	Unengaged by issue	Never thought about testing	Do not plan to test in next 6 months	
	↓	↓	↓	Contemplation
Stage 3	Deciding about acting	Undecided about testing	Plan to test in next 6 months	↓
Stage 4	↑ Decided not to act	→ Decided not to test		
	↓	↓	↓	Preparation
Stage 5	Decided to act	Decided to test	Plan to test in next 3 months	↓
	↓	↓	↓	Action
Stage 6	Acting	Testing	Testing	↓
	↓	↓	↓	Maintenance
Stage 7	Maintenance	Not applicable	Not applicable	

Figure 4.1 Comparison of the Precaution Adoption Process Model and the Transtheoretical Model

Note: The precontemplation, contemplation and preparation stages of the Transtheoretical Model are not aligned with the first three stages of the Precaution Process Model because these two sets of stages are not equivalent. Note that the preparation stage of the Transtheoretical Model usually has a second requirement, that the person has made a previous attempt to carry out the action within the past year. Since with this requirement no one can get to the preparation stage for a first attempt, such a formulation of the model would obviously be appropriate only if everyone had already attempted the action in the past.

1992). The PAPM identifies seven stages along the path from ignorance to action. At some initial point in time people are unaware of the health issue (Stage 1). When they first learn something about the issue, they are no longer unaware, but they are not necessarily engaged by it either (Stage 2). People who reach the decision-making stage (Stage 3) have become engaged by the issue and are considering their response. This decision-making process can result in one of two outcomes. If the decision is not to take any action, the precaution adoption process ends (Stage 4), at least for the time being. But if people decide to adopt the precaution (Stage 5), the next step is to initiate the behaviour (Stage 6). A seventh stage, if appropriate, indicates that the behaviour has been maintained over time (Stage 7).

The PAPM has been applied to osteoporosis prevention (Blalock *et al.* 1996), mammography (Clemow *et al.* 2000), hepatitis B vaccination (Hammer 1997) and home radon testing (Weinstein and Sandman 1992; Weinstein *et al.* 1998a). The stages in radon testing suggested by the model are shown in Figure 4.1. (Although repeat radon testing is recommended by experts under some circumstances, radon testing is still largely a one-time process. Therefore, the maintenance phase is not shown in the figure.)

The model asserts that people usually pass through the stages in sequence, without skipping any, though there is no minimum length of time that must be spent in any one stage. Movement backwards towards an earlier stage can also occur, without necessarily going through all the intermediate stages, though obviously it is not possible to go from later stages to Stages 1 or 2.

The PAPM appears similar to another stage theory, the Transtheoretical Model (TTM) developed by Prochaska, DiClemente, Velicer and their colleagues (Prochaska and DiClemente 1983; Velicer *et al.* 1985; DiClemente *et al.* 1991; Prochaska *et al.* 1991; Prochaska and DiClemente 1992). A glance at Figure 4.1, however, shows that most of the similarities are superficial, reflecting the names that have been given to the stages rather than the actual way in which the stages are defined. For example, the PAPM distinguishes among people who are unaware of an issue (Stage 1), those who know something about an issue but have never actively thought about it (Stage 2) and those who have decided not to adopt the precaution (Stage 4). In the TTM, all are grouped together in the precontemplation stage. Studies comparing people in Stages 2 and 4 of the PAPM find considerable differences between the two groups (Weinstein and Sandman 1992; Blalock *et al.* 1996).

A second difference between the PAPM and the TTM concerns the criteria used to assign people to stages. The stages of the TTM are based on two variables: past behaviour (whether or not the individual has tried to carry out the behaviour in the past) and the length of time before they intend to try again. Assignment to PAPM stages is based solely on a person's current thoughts about the behaviour, without reliance on any particular time frame.

2.2 Justification for the PAPM stages

There should be good reasons for proposing the separate stages in a stage model. What is the justification for the stages of the PAPM?

Stage 1 (Unaware)

Much health research deals with well-known hazards, like smoking and AIDS. In such cases, asking someone about their beliefs and plans is quite reasonable, since most people have thought about the relevance of these threats to their own lives. But if people have never heard of a hazard, they certainly have no opinions about it. The reluctance of respondents to answer survey questions about less familiar issues suggests that investigators ought to allow people to say that they 'don't know' or have 'no opinion' rather than forcing them to state a position. Participants in health behaviour research are seldom given this opportunity.

Stage 2 (Unengaged) versus Stage 3 (Deciding about acting)

Once people have heard about a hazard and have begun to form opinions about it, they are no longer in Stage 1. However, so many issues compete for our limited time and attention that people can know a fair amount about a hazard yet never have considered whether they need to do anything about it. We believe that this condition of awareness without personal engagement is quite common. In a 1986 survey of radon testing (Weinstein *et al.* 1987), for example, 50 per cent of respondents in a high-risk region said that they had never thought about testing their own homes; all had previously indicated that they knew what radon was.

The PAPM suggests further that it is important to distinguish between the people who have never thought about an action and those who have given the action some consideration but are undecided. For example, attitudes based on personal experience with an issue are more predictive of future behaviour than attitudes generated on the spot, without such experience (Fazio and Zanna 1981). Thus, whether a person has or has not seen an issue as requiring a personal decision appears to be an important distinction.

Stage 3 (Deciding about acting) versus Stage 4 (Decided not to act) and Stage 5 (Decided to act)

Research reveals important differences between people who have not yet formed an opinion and those who have come to a decision. People who have come to a definite position on an issue – especially an issue regarding their own behaviour – have different responses to information and are more resistant to persuasion than people who have never formed an opinion (Nisbett and Ross 1980: ch. 8; Anderson 1983; Jelalian and Miller 1984; Brockner and Rubin 1985; Cialdini 1988). Thus, it is significant when people say that they have decided to act, and saying they have decided to act is not the same as saying it is 'very likely' they will act.

One variable that frequently differentiates among people who have decided to act, those who are undecided, and those who have decided not to act is perceived susceptibility (also called 'perceived personal likelihood'). This factor is included in most theories of health behaviour (Conner and Norman 1996). Since people are reluctant to acknowledge personal susceptibility to harm even when they acknowledge the risk faced by others (Weinstein 1987), it appears that overcoming this reluctance is one of the barriers to getting people to decide to act.

Stage 5 (Decided to act) versus Stage 6 (Acting)
The distinction between decision and action is not an original idea. Ajzen's Theory of Planned Behaviour (Ajzen 1985; Ajzen and Madden 1986), for example, distinguishes between intentions and action. A growing body of research (Gollwitzer 1999) suggests that there are important gaps between intending to act and carrying out this intention and that helping people develop implementation plans can reduce these barriers. Detailed implementation information that would be uninteresting to people in earlier stages may be essential at this transition.

Stage 6 (Acting) versus Stage 7 (Maintenance)
The distinction between action and maintenance is widely recognized (for example Marlatt and Gordon 1985; Meichanbaum and Turk 1987; Dishman 1988) and will not be discussed here. Suggestions about other factors that may be important at different transitions are given in Weinstein (1988).

3 The intervention

A field experiment focusing on radon testing was designed to examine several aspects of the PAPM. The main features of the experiment are described here both to indicate how experiments with stage theories can be constructed and analysed and to communicate the results of the experiment. Additional details are available elsewhere (Weinstein *et al.* 1998a).

The experiment focused on two stage transitions: from being undecided about testing one's home for radon (Stage 3) to deciding to test (Stage 5), and from deciding to test (Stage 5) to actually ordering a test (Stage 6). The study did not look at the transition from being unaware of the radon issue (Stage 1) to being aware but not engaged (Stage 2), or from being unengaged (Stage 2) to thinking about testing (Stage 3), because merely agreeing to participate in a radon study and answering questions about testing would probably be sufficient to produce these changes. People who had already decided not to test (Stage 4) were excluded because a brief intervention would probably be unable to reverse that decision.

To determine whether the two transitions studied involve different barriers, as the theory claims, two interventions were needed, one matched to each transition. Previous surveys and experiments (Weinstein *et al.* 1990; Sandman and Weinstein 1993) gave insights into the potential barriers. They suggested that increasing homeowners' perceptions of their own risk – that is, increasing the perceived likelihood of having unhealthy radon levels in their homes – is important in getting undecided people to decide to test. This was chosen as the goal of one intervention.

Interventions focusing on risk had not been effective, however, in getting people actually to order tests (Weinstein *et al.* 1990, 1991). Instead, several studies had found that test orders could be increased by increasing the ease of testing (Weinstein *et al.* 1990, 1991; Doyle *et al.* 1991). Thus, for people who had already decided to test, the second intervention was intended to reduce barriers to action by providing information about do-it-yourself test kits and a test order form.

3.1 Method

Study design

The study took place in Columbus, Ohio, a city with high radon levels. Since the issue had received hardly any attention for several years, we were concerned that homeowners' thoughts about testing might be weakly held and that any stage assessment would be unstable. Consequently, all participants viewed a general informational video before receiving any experimental treatment. Their stage of testing was assessed after this first video (preintervention measurement).

After the questionnaire had been returned and eligibility to continue had been ascertained, the experimental videos were delivered to participants. One intervention (High-Likelihood) focused on increasing the perceived likelihood of having a home radon problem. The second (Low-Effort) focused on decreasing the perceived and actual effort required to test. These two treatments were combined factorially to create four conditions: Control (no intervention), High-Likelihood, Low-Effort, and Combination (High-Likelihood + Low-Effort). Stage of testing was assessed immediately after the experimental treatment (post-intervention measurement) and several months later.

Intervention videos

Three different videos were developed for the experiment. All participants viewed a six-minute tape entitled *Basic Facts about Radon*, which provided an overview of the topic but included only general information about radon risk and testing procedures.

The High-Likelihood treatment consisted of a five-minute video, *Radon Risk in Columbus Area Homes*, and a covering letter. The goal of the video was to convince people that they had a moderate to high chance of finding unhealthy radon levels in their own homes. Results of radon studies indicating high local levels, pictures of actual local homes with high levels, and testimony by a local homeowner and a city health official all presented evidence of the problem. Myths about radon levels that had been identified in past research were presented and refuted. The covering letter mentioned that test kits could be ordered from the American Lung Association (ALA), but did not include an order form.

Participants in the Low-Effort condition received a five-minute video, *How to Test your Home for Radon*, a covering letter and a form to order test kits through the ALA. The video described how to select a kit type (making an explicit recommendation in order to reduce uncertainty), locate and purchase a kit, and conduct a test. The process was represented as simple and inexpensive.

Participants in the Combination condition received a ten-minute video that was simply the combination of the two separate treatments. They received the same letter and order form as people in the Low-Effort condition.

Participants in the Control condition received a letter stating that their assistance in viewing a second video was not needed (recall that they had already viewed *Basic Facts about Radon*) and mentioning that test kits could be ordered from the ALA.

Procedure

Study participants were initially contacted by telephone. Those homeowners who had at least heard of radon, who had not tested and who agreed to take part (n = 4706) were mailed the video, *Basic Facts about Radon*, and a questionnaire assessing their reactions. The particular question designed to assess stage of testing asked 'What are your thoughts about testing your home for radon?' The choices offered were 'I have already completed a test, have a test in progress, or have purchased a test' (Stage 6); 'I have never thought about testing my home' (Stage 2); 'I'm undecided about testing' (Stage 3); 'I've decided I *don't* want to test' (Stage 4); and 'I've decided I *do* want to test' (Stage 5).

Those individuals who were either in the 'undecided' stage or 'decided to test' stage after watching *Basic Facts about Radon* were assigned at random to one of the four experimental conditions and were mailed the intervention materials appropriate for that condition and a feedback questionnaire. To enhance the impact of the interventions, participants were asked to watch each video twice, once for content and once for style. The response rate to the second video was 73.2 per cent, with no significant differences among conditions.

Follow-up telephone interviews (completion rate = 94.5 per cent) were carried out 9–10 weeks after respondents returned the second video questionnaire. These asked whether participants had purchased a radon test kit and, if not, determined their final stage.

3.2 Results

The final sample consisted of 1897 homeowners. After watching *Basic Facts about Radon*, the division among stages of those retained in the study was 28.8 per cent 'undecided' and 71.2 per cent 'decided-to-test'.

Manipulation checks based on items in the questionnaires verified that the High-Likelihood intervention had succeeded in substantially increasing perceived risk and that the Low-Effort intervention had succeeded in convincing people that testing is easy. The Combination intervention accomplished both these goals, with no evidence that its impacts on these beliefs were anything other than the additive effects of its separate components.

Predicting progress towards action

Table 4.1 shows the percentage of people from each preintervention stage who progressed *one or more* stages towards testing. This criterion (rather than progress of only one stage towards testing) was chosen because, although people who had been stopped at one stage were hypothesized to lack the requirements to get to the next stage, there was no a priori reason to assume that they did not already possess the information or skills needed to overcome later barriers. The upper half of the table indicates the percentage of people at follow-up who had moved from the undecided stage to either the decided-to-test or the testing stage. The lower half of the table shows the percentage of decided-to-test people who had moved on to the testing stage.

Statistical analyses showed more people progressing from the undecided stage than from the decided-to-test stage, $F(1, 1886) = 61.6$, $p < 0.0001$, and more progress from those who received the High-Likelihood treatment than from those who did not, $F(1, 1886) = 31.5$, $p < 0.0001$. Most importantly, as expected from the use of matched and mismatched interventions,

Table 4.1   Progressed one or more stage towards purchasing a radon test (%)

	Condition			
Preintervention stage	Control	High-Likelihood	Low-Effort	Combination
Undecided	18.8 (138)	41.7 (144)	36.4 (130)	54.5 (139)
Decided-to-test	8.0 (339)	10.4 (338)	32.5 (329)	35.8 (345)

Note: The group size in each cell is shown in parentheses

there was a significant stage by High-Likelihood Treatment interaction, $F(1, 1886) = 18.5$, $p < 0.0001$, indicating that the High-Likelihood treatment was much more effective for undecided participants than for decided-to-act participants.

There was also a large main effect of the Low-Effort treatment, $F(1, 1886) = 89.4$, $p < 0.0001$. The stage by Low-Effort treatment interaction, $F(1, 1886) = 5.9$, $p < 0.02$, indicated that, as hypothesized, the Low-Effort treatment in the Low-Effort and Combination conditions had a relatively bigger effect on people already planning to test than on people who were undecided. The High-Likelihood by Low-Effort interaction and the three-way interaction were not significant.

Predicting test orders
The follow-up interviews revealed that radon tests were ordered by 342 study participants or 18.0 per cent of the sample. The data concerning test orders are presented in Table 4.2. For people initially planning to test, 'progress' and testing are the same according to the PAPM, so the data in the lower half of Table 4.2 are identical to those in the lower half of Table 4.1. As expected, there was more testing from the decided-to-test stage than from the undecided stage, $F(1, 1887) = 42.3$, $p < 0.0001$. In addition, there was much more testing from people exposed to a Low-Effort treatment than from those who did not receive this treatment, $F(1, 1887) = 87.9$, $p < 0.0001$. The High-Likelihood treatment effect and the Low-Effort by High-Likelihood interaction were not significant, p's > 0.1 Most important was the highly significant interaction between stage and Low-Effort treatment, $F(1, 1887) = 18.2$, $p < 0.0001$. The other interactions (stage by High-Likelihood and stage by Low-Effort by High-Likelihood) were not significant (p's > 0.1).

More specific tests concern predicted cell-by-cell contrasts. In subsequent paragraphs the predictions are presented in brackets and experimental groups are labelled with letters that refer to the cells in Table 4.2.

Test order rates of both undecided and decided-to-test participants in the Control condition were expected to be quite low since both groups were viewed as lacking information needed to progress to action [(a) ≈ (e),

Table 4.2   Radon test orders (%)

Preintervention stage	Condition			
	Control	High-Likelihood	Low-Effort	Combination
Undecided	(a) 5.1	(b) 3.5	(c) 10.1	(d) 18.7
Decided-to-test	(e) 8.0	(f) 10.4	(g) 32.5	(h) 35.8

both small]. The main problems facing people who had decided to test were hypothesized to be the difficulties in choosing, purchasing and using radon test kits. Thus, the Low-Effort treatment was expected to be much more helpful than the high-risk treatment in getting people in this stage to order tests [(g) > (f)]. In fact, past research (Weinstein *et al.* 1990, 1991) suggested that the High-Likelihood treatment would be ineffective in eliciting testing from people planning to test [(f) ≈ (e)], and, more obviously, would be unable to elicit test orders from undecided people [(b) ≈ (a)]. Furthermore, since it was anticipated that people in the decided-to-test stage did not need further information about risk, we predicted that testing in the Combination condition would not be significantly greater than testing in the Low-Effort condition [(h) ≈ (g)].

According to the PAPM, people who are undecided have to decide to test before acting, so a Low-Effort intervention alone was not expected to produce test orders from this group [(c) ≈ (a)]. However, undecided people in the Combination condition received both high-likelihood information (seen as important in deciding to test) and low-effort assistance (seen as important for carrying out action intentions). Some of these people might be able to make two stage transitions [(d) > (c)], but not as many as decided-to-test people in the Combination condition who needed to advance only one stage [(d) < (h)].

T-tests comparing the means of the cells mentioned in the preceding eight hypotheses demonstrated that none of the pairs predicted to be approximately the same were significantly different (p's > 0.3), but all pairs predicted to be different were significantly different (all p's < 0.0001 except for the hypothesis that (d) > (c), p = 0.03).

Further calculations of two-stage transitions

The cell-by-cell predictions just examined were based on the expectation that the interventions would be completely stage-specific, a somewhat unrealistic expectation. In particular, our initial prediction about the rate of testing from undecided people in the Low-Effort condition (cell c) was based on the expectation that this treatment would not persuade anyone that they should test. Yet Table 4.1 shows that the Low-Effort treatment did get many undecided people to decide to test. Given this new knowledge, how should we revise our predictions?

According to the Precaution Adoption Process Model, in order to test, undecided people have to make two separate stage transitions. If these transitions are viewed as independent, sequential steps, the probability of a person moving forward two steps (from undecided to testing) should be the product of the two separate probabilities involved: the probability that undecided people move towards testing (and thus get at least to the decided-to-test stage) times the probability that people who get to the decided-to-test stage carry out this decision. According to this reasoning, the predicted rate of testing by undecided people in the Low-Effort condition should be $0.364 \times 0.325 = 0.118$ or 11.8 per cent (see Table 4.1). This is very close to the observed value of 10.1 per cent in Table 4.2. This same argument can be used to calculate testing rates for undecided people in the Combination condition. The expected rate of testing in this cell is $0.545 \times 0.358 = 0.195$ or 19.5 per cent. This is again extremely close to the observed value of 18.7 per cent in Table 4.2.

4 Discussion: implications for theory, policy and practice

4.1 Implications for theory

The results of the study just discussed have obvious theoretical implications. They provide support for our claim that never having thought about an action, being undecided, and having decided to act represent distinct stages, with different barriers between stages. The data also support the suggestion that information about risk is helpful in getting people to decide to act, even though this same information may have little value in producing action among those individuals who have already decided to act. Furthermore, information that increases the perceived and actual ease of action appears to greatly aid people who have decided to test, but it is relatively less important among people who are still undecided. Obviously, more research is needed to test whether these same factors are important at the same stages for other health behaviours.

Acceptance of the idea that stages exist also has implications for theory development in general. If the factors facilitating movement towards action vary from stage to stage, few if any factors will be important at all stages. Thus, comparing two groups of people, those who have acted and all others who have not acted, is likely to be a poor strategy for discovering variables important for precaution adoption. A variable may be a powerful determinant of progress at one particular stage, but it may look rather weak if actors are compared with everyone else. Stage theories suggest that we will be better able to recognize important issues if we compare people who are in adjacent stages.

4.2 Implications for policy and practice

The results of the radon testing experiment are big enough to have practical implications. When viewed in terms of odds ratios – for example, the three-fold difference in test orders between the undecided and decided-to-test stages in the Low-Effort condition or the tenfold difference between cells with the highest and lowest testing rates – the effects observed were quite large.

Stage-targeted communications have never been used in actual radon testing promotions, and until recently have not been used for any health behaviours. The most widely disseminated radon communications, national television public service advertisements, focused on persuading viewers that the radon hazard is substantial for people in general. To the extent that a target audience stage can be inferred, these public service advertisements appeared to be aimed primarily at viewers who were unaware of the radon problem (Stage 1) or had never thought about their own response (Stage 2). This was a defensible choice when the issue was new and the medium used (national television) was scattershot. But 15 years after radon started to receive substantial public attention, most radon communication campaigns have retained the same focus, even though the media available permit greater specificity and there is reason to think that much of the audience is beyond Stages 1 and 2.

4.3 Criteria for applying stage-based interventions

As the preceding paragraph implies, a variety of issues need to be considered to determine the practical utility of the PAPM or of any other stage model.

Superiority over unstaged messages

The practical utility of a stage model obviously depends on the extent to which it leads to interventions that are more effective than generic messages for people at particular stages. For the radon testing study described here we developed two different interventions. The interventions chosen were based on years of research and experience on radon testing in general, plus an elaborate pilot project in the target community.

As predicted, individual vulnerability turned out to be a particularly useful message for people in the Columbus area at the undecided stage of the radon testing decision. We suggested that vulnerability is always (or usually) a key issue for transitions from Stage 3 to Stage 5 – as opposed to, say, information about illness severity – but this suggestion requires verification. Ease of testing turned out to be particularly useful to those Columbus residents who had already decided to test but had not yet done so. We suggested that detailed instructions for carrying out precautions information is key to transitions from Stage 5 to Stage 6, but this idea also needs testing. Yet even if a stage theory does not specify all the barriers between each pair of stages, it may, if it correctly categorizes people facing similar obstacles, help in the discovery of what those obstacles are.

Since the combination treatment in our experiment produced the greatest progress among both undecided and decided-to-test participants, one might be tempted to conclude that the PAPM did not provide any new treatment ideas. 'Just use the combination treatment', someone might say. There are several flaws in this reasoning. First, it is important to recall that the combination treatment was approximately twice as long as each of its two components. Media time is expensive; speakers usually have a fixed length of time for their presentations; audiences have a limited attention span. Thus, attempting to replace the Low-Effort or High-Likelihood interventions with their combination would involve substantial costs. Second, although no evidence is available on this point, people seem likely to be more engaged by a treatment that matches their stage. For example, unlike people participating in a research study, members of the general public who are undecided about taking a precaution may not pay attention to the detailed procedural information they might need later to carry out that precaution. Third, among people who had decided to act, risk information was superfluous. Nevertheless, if only a single message can be given to a mixed-stage audience, the combination intervention would probably be the most appropriate.

Stage assessment
A second relevant criterion is the ability to identify stages accurately and efficiently. The PAPM requires only a single question to assess a person's stage, so it can be used easily in individual or small-group settings. Even in a large audience, a show of hands could be quickly used to determine the distribution of stages present, though this would be inappropriate if the topic under discussion were sensitive. However, if the audience is dispersed and the budget is small or time is tight, efforts to measure stage may be impractical. Furthermore, a single assessment may not be enough. Progress towards action may need to be monitored over time so that the interventions or messages can change to match the current stages of the intended audience.

Also requiring consideration is the accuracy and reliability of stage assessments, since in all current stage theories these are based on self reports. These factors are likely to depend on the frequency and recency with which audience members have considered the health topic. When people are asked about new hazards or new precautions or about old ones that they have not thought about for years, their responses may be unreliable and tell us little about their actions or concerns. Essentially nothing is known about factors determining the accuracy of stage assessments. People, for example, might overstate their interest in actions that are socially desirable, possibly making a written assessment method superior to a verbal assessment.

Delivery of targeted messages
The feasibility of delivering stage-targeted messages in different situations varies greatly. If communication is one-to-one, as in a doctor's surgery or counselling session, delivering the message appropriate for the individual is quite easy. In group settings, such as public lectures, messages can be chosen to fit the overall audience, though not individual members. In mass communications a stage approach is more often useful with print than with

broadcast media. Within print, pamphlets and magazines offer more opportunities for stage targeting than newspapers; within broadcasting, cable
offers more opportunities for stage targeting than networks.

A closely related question is the browsability or searchability of the
medium. Although we tend to think of targeting as something the communicator does, audience members can also 'target' the content they need.
The more browsable and searchable a medium, the easier it is for each
audience member to seek out content appropriate to their stage. A lecture,
video tape or broadcast programme is extremely low on this dimension.
Whatever comes next comes next, and the audience's only choice is whether
to continue listening. By contrast, print messages are much more browsable/
searchable, and well-designed aids such as subheads and indexes take advantage of this capacity. The Internet and interactive computer programs are
more browsable/searchable still. If each audience member can be relied
upon to find the most stage-relevant information, it may be possible to reap
the advantages of stage targeting without actually having to target, simply
by facilitating audience self-targeting. Of course this is not just a matter of
choosing and using the medium wisely. Self-targeting takes motivation.
Audiences to whom the issue is hot probably will seek out what they need
to know (or at least what they think they need to know). Audiences for whom
the issue is either unfamiliar or boringly familiar probably will not.

The ability to deliver targeted messages to members of a group also
depends on the range of stages present in that group. The greater the range
of stages present, the more difficult it is to choose a single message. For a
mass audience, the most efficient way to encourage a new health-protective
action may be with a comprehensive broadcast message that ignores stage
or assumes everyone to be at a very early stage. As the issue matures, however, distinctive audiences, separable by stage, merit distinctive messages,
and print or 'narrowcasting' becomes the medium of choice for mass communications. Thus, stage-based messages are likely to be more important
for relatively mature health issues than for emerging ones.

Difficulty of behaviour change
A final criterion of importance concerns the difficulty of the health behaviour being advocated and the expected audience resistance to the message.
When the behaviour is easy and resistance is low, stage matters less. With
such behaviours, the interventions or messages needed to help people progress from stage to stage may be brief. Several may be combined into a single
comprehensive treatment. When change is difficult and resistance is high, in
contrast, there is a greater need for the delivery of separate messages for
each stage.

In the radon testing study, the general, preintervention video tape moved
many participants through several stages. At recruitment, only 8 per cent of
participants said that they had decided to test, but after the preintervention

video over 70 per cent said they had decided to test, including many who had said initially that they had never thought about testing (and thus moved two stages). Similarly, the Low-Effort intervention persuaded many undecided people to order tests. We can imagine study participants who were reluctant to test nevertheless telling themselves 'If it is really that simple and inexpensive, I might as well do it' – in effect skipping the decision-making process on the grounds that such a low-effort behaviour was easier to implement than to evaluate. Radon testing is so easy, and radon test kits so accessible, that it comes as a surprise to many professionals that there is any need for the Low-Effort intervention. Most other health behaviours are not nearly so easy, and many audiences are not nearly so unresisting. In such cases, stage targeting would be expected to matter more.

Clearly, stage-based targeted interventions are more complex, and thus usually more expensive, than standardized, one-size-fits-all interventions. They may be more complex and expensive than targeted interventions based on psychological or demographic distinctions other than stages. Thus, it seems likely that there will be situations where the improvement in the stage-based intervention's performance is not large enough to justify its use. Nevertheless, there are numerous health behaviours that have proved resistant to standard health promotion approaches. Examples include car seatbelt use, weight loss, smoking prevention and condom use. Although the extra cost of stage approaches must be weighed against the extra benefit they may provide, many already tried interventions have had such limited success that whether they offer any benefit at all is questionable. In such situations, the need to try new approaches seems undeniable.

Acknowledgements

The authors are indebted to Alexander Rothman and Stephen Sutton for their assistance in clarifying the characteristics and testing of stage theories and to Cara Cuite, May Lou Klotz, Judith Lyon and Nancy Roberts for their contributions to our radon research. Funding for the radon research from the New Jersey Department of Environmental Protection, the New Jersey Agricultural Experiment Station and the National Cancer Institute is gratefully acknowledged.

References

Ajzen, I. (1985) From intentions to actions: a theory of planned behaviour, in J. Kuhl and J. Beckman (eds) *Action Control: From Cognition to Behaviour*. Heidelberg: Springer.

Ajzen, I. and Fishbein, M. (eds) (1980) *Understanding Attitudes and Predicting Social Behavior*. Englewood Cliffs, NJ: Prentice-Hall.

Ajzen, I. and Madden, T.J. (1986) Prediction of goal-directed behavior: attitudes, intention, and perceived behavioral control, *Journal of Experimental Social Psychology*, 22: 453–74.

Anderson, C.A. (1983) Abstract and concrete data in the perseverance of social theories: when weak data lead to unshakable beliefs, *Journal of Experimental Social Psychology*, 19: 93–108.

Bandura, A. (1995) Moving into forward gear in health promotion and disease prevention. Address presented at the annual meeting of the Society of Behavioral Medicine, San Diego, CA, March.

Blalock, S.J., DeVellis, R.F., Giorgino, K.B. *et al.* (1996) Osteoporosis prevention in premenopausal women: using a stage model approach to examine the predictors of behavior, *Health Psychology*, 15(2): 84–93.

Brockner, J. and Rubin, J.Z. (1985) *Entrapment in Escalating Conflicts: A Social Psychological Analysis*. New York: Springer.

Cialdini, R.B. (1988) *Influence: Theory and Practice*. Glenview, IL: Scott, Foresman.

Clemow, L., Costanza, M.E., Haddad, W.P. *et al.* (2000) Underutilizers of mammography screening today: characteristics of women planning, undecided about, and not planning a mammogram, *Annals of Behavioral Medicine*, 22(1): 80–8.

Conner, M. and Norman, P. (eds) (1996) *Predicting Health Behaviour: Research and Practice with Social Cognition Models*. Buckingham: Open University Press.

DiClemente, C.C., Prochaska, J.O., Fairhurst, S.K. *et al.* (1991) The process of smoking cessation: an analysis of precontemplation, contemplation, and preparation stages of change, *Journal of Consulting and Clinical Psychology*, 59: 295–304.

Dishman, R.K. (1988) *Exercise Adherence: Its Impact on Public Health*. Champaign, IL: Human Kinetics.

Doyle, J.K., McClelland, G.H. and Schulze, W.D. (1991) Protective responses to household risk: a case study of radon mitigation, *Risk Analysis*, 11: 121–34.

Edwards, W. (1954) The theory of decision making, *Psychological Bulletin*, 51: 380–417.

Fazio, R.H. and Zanna, M.P. (1981) Direct experience and attitude–behavior consistency, in L. Berkowitz (ed.) *Advances in Experimental Social Psychology* 14. New York: Academic Press.

Fishbein, M. and Ajzen, I. (1975) *Belief, Attitude, Intention and Behavior: An Introduction to Theory and Research*. Reading, MA: Addison-Wesley.

Fishbein, M. and Middlestadt, S.E. (1989) Using the theory of reasoned action as a framework for understanding and changing AIDS-related behaviors, in V.M. Mays, G.W. Albee and S.F. Schneider (eds) *Primary Prevention of AIDS: Psychological Approaches*. Newbury Park, CA: Sage.

Gollwitzer, P.M. (1999) Implementation intentions: strong effects of simple plans, *American Psychologist*, 54(7): 493–503.

Hammer, G.P. (1997) Hepatitis B vaccine acceptance among nursing home workers. Unpublished dissertation, Department of Health Policy and Management, Johns Hopkins University, Baltimore, MD.

Hedeker, D., Mermelstein, R.J. and Weeks, K.A. (1999) The thresholds of change model: an approach to analyzing stages of change data, *Annals of Behavioral Medicine*, 21: 61–70.

Janz, N. and Becker, M.H. (1984) The health belief model: a decade later, *Health Education Quarterly*, 11: 1–47.

Jelalian, E. and Miller, A.G. (1984) The perseverance of beliefs: conceptual perspectives and research developments, *Journal of Social and Clinical Psychology*, 2: 25–56.

Kirscht, J.P. (1988) The health belief model and predictions of health actions, in D. Gochman (ed.) *Health Behavior*. New York: Plenum.

Marlatt, G.A. and Gordon, J.R. (1985) *Relapse Prevention: Maintenance Strategies in the Treatment of Addictive Behaviors*. New York: Guilford.

Meichanbaum, D. and Turk, D.C. (1987) *Facilitating Treatment Adherence: A Practitioner's Handbook*. New York: Plenum.

Nisbett, R. and Ross, L. (1980) *Human Inference: Strategies and Shortcomings of Social Judgment*. Englewood Cliffs, NJ: Prentice-Hall.

Prentice-Dunn, S. and Rogers, R.W. (1986) Protection motivation theory and preventive health: beyond the health belief model, *Health Education Research*, 1(3): 153–61.

Prochaska, J.O. and DiClemente, C.C. (1983) Stages and processes of self-change in smoking: toward an integrative model of change, *Journal of Consulting and Clinical Psychology*, 51: 390–5.

Prochaska, J.O. and DiClemente, C.C. (1992) Stages of change in the modification of problem behaviors, in M. Hersen, R.M. Eisler and P.M. Miller (eds) *Progress in Behavior Modification*, 28. Sycamore, IL: Sycamore Publishing Co.

Prochaska, J.O., Velicer, W.F., DiClemente, C.C., Guadagnoli, E. and Rossi, J.S. (1991) Patterns of change: dynamic typology applied to smoking cessation, *Multivariate Behavioral Research*, 26: 83–107.

Rogers, R.W. (1983) Cognitive and physiological processes in fear appeals and attitude change, in J.T. Cacioppo and R.E. Petty (eds) *Social Psychophysiology*. New York: Guilford.

Ronis, D.L. (1992) Conditional health threats: health beliefs, decisions, and behaviors among adults, *Health Psychology*, 11: 127–34.

Rosenstock, I.M. (1974) The health belief model: origins and correlates, *Health Education Monographs*, 2: 36–353.

Sandman, P.M. and Weinstein, N.D. (1993) Predictors of home radon testing and implications for testing promotion programs, *Health Education Quarterly*, 20: 1–17.

Sutton, S.R. (1982) Fear arousing communications: a critical examination of theory and research, in J.R. Eiser (ed.) *Social Psychology and Behavioral Medicine*. New York: Wiley.

US Environmental Protection Agency Office of Radiation Programs (1991) *National Residential Radon Survey: Statistical Analysis, National and Regional Estimates*, Volume I. Washington, DC: Author.

US Environmental Protection Agency Office of Radiation Programs (1992) *Technical Support Document for the Citizen's Guide to Radon (EPA 400-R-92-011)*. Washington, DC: Author.

US Environmental Protection Agency Office of Radiation Programs and US Department of Health and Human Services Centers for Disease Control (1992) *A Citizen's Guide to Radon*, 2nd edn. Washington, DC: Author.

US National Academy of Sciences (1988) *Health Effects of Radon and Other Internally Deposited Alpha-Emitters: BEIR IV*. Washington, DC: National Academy Press.

Velicer, W.F., DiClemente, C.C., Prochaska, J.O. and Brandenburg, N. (1985) Decisional balance measure for assessing and predicting smoking status, *Journal of Personality and Social Psychology*, 48, 1279–89.

Weinstein, N.D. (1987) Unrealistic optimism about susceptibility to health problems: conclusions from a community-wide sample, *Journal of Behavioural Medicine*, 10: 481–500.

Weinstein, N.D. (1988) The precaution adoption process, *Health Psychology*, 7(4): 355–86.

Weinstein, N.D. (1993) Testing four competing theories of health-protective behaviour, *Health Psychology*, 12(4): 324–33.

Weinstein, N.D. and Sandman, P.M. (1992) A model of the precaution adoption process: evidence from home radon testing, *Health Psychology*, 11(3): 170–80.

Weinstein, N.D., Lyon, J.E., Sandman, P.M. and Cuite, C.L. (1998a) Experimental evidence for stages of health behavior change: the precaution adoption process model applied to home radon testing, *Health Psychology*, 17(5): 445–53.

Weinstein, N.D., Rothman, A.J. and Sutton, S.R. (1998b) Stage theories of health behavior: conceptual and methodological issues, *Health Psychology*, 17(3): 290–9.

Weinstein, N.D., Sandman, P.M. and Klotz, M.L. (1987) *Public Response to the Risk from Radon, 1986*. New Brunswick, NJ: Environmental Communications Research Program, Rutgers University.

Weinstein, N.D., Sandman, P.M. and Roberts, N.E. (1990) Determinants of self-protective behavior: home radon testing, *Journal of Applied Social Psychology*, 20: 783–801.

Weinstein, N.D., Sandman, P.M. and Roberts, N.E. (1991) Perceived susceptibility and self-protective behavior: a field experiment to encourage home radon testing, *Health Psychology*, 10: 25–33.

| 5 | CHRISTOPHER J. ARMITAGE |
| | AND MARK CONNER |

REDUCING FAT INTAKE: INTERVENTIONS BASED ON THE THEORY OF PLANNED BEHAVIOUR

This chapter presents a Theory of Planned Behaviour-based intervention designed to reduce fat intake. The first section reviews the evidence surrounding the diet–health relationship, focusing on the effects of excessive fat consumption. The second section presents the Theory of Planned Behaviour (Ajzen 1991) as a model for developing theory-based interventions. The third section reports a study that utilizes the TPB to inform a dietary intervention. The final section discusses ways in which the present findings may be extended.

1 Reducing fat intake

1.1 The link between diet and health

A considerable body of work documents the close link between dietary intake and health. Dietary factors have been implicated in the aetiology of a number of serious conditions, including several cancers, cardiovascular diseases, hypertension and diabetes. Cancer and coronary heart disease in particular represent the leading causes of death in industrialized countries, and account for a large proportion of health expenditure. Government-level response to this has focused on the setting of dietary targets to promote health (for example US Department of Health and Human Services 1991; Department of Health 1992). These guidelines provide recommended daily intakes of food by nutrient group, and encompass salt intake, fat intake, fruit and vegetable intake, and fibre intake. This chapter focuses on reducing fat intake.

Excessive fat intake has been particularly closely linked with increased morbidity and mortality from a number of serious conditions, including coronary heart disease and cancer (for example Temple 1996; Trichopoulos and Willett 1996). The UK government recommends that no more than 35 per cent of food energy should be derived from fat in the diet, and no more than 11 per cent from saturated fat (Department of Health 1992). Recent trends suggest this target is unlikely to be reached in the near future: fat intake as a proportion of total calorific intake has remained at 40 per cent since the 1970s and 1980s (Ministry of Agriculture, Fisheries and Food (MAFF) 1992).[1]

The increased risk of coronary heart disease and cancer associated with excessive fat intake derives from increased levels of low density lipoproteins in serum, which are assumed to increase as a function of saturated fat intake (for example Stallones 1983). Although the evidence that directly links dietary fat intake with blood cholesterol level is not as strong as is often assumed (Stallones 1983), there are other benefits to be derived from reducing fat consumption. Evidence suggests that fat intake is the most important determinant of overall energy intake: Westerterp *et al.* (1996) showed that over six months, fat intake accounted for 70 per cent of the variance in change in energy intake. Therefore, reducing fat intake will have a proportionately greater impact on weight reduction, compared with reduced intake of other macronutrients. Given that obesity and being overweight *per se* have been associated with a wide range of conditions, including cardiovascular diseases, arthritis and non-insulin dependent diabetes (for example Oomura *et al.* 1991), there are clear benefits to be derived from attempts to reduce fat intake.

1.2 Dietary interventions

Intensive dietary interventions targeted at individuals deemed to be 'at risk' have generally been successful in reducing fat intake (Schapira *et al.* 1991). However, by definition, such approaches require time and resources, and focus only on 'at-risk' individuals. An attractive alternative is the use of large-scale public health messages aimed at the general population. Evidence for the utility of these approaches has been equivocal (MAFF 1992; Family Heart Study Group 1994; OXCHECK Study Group 1994); even where positive effects have been observed, there have been few attempts to examine the role of potential mediating variables (for example Maccoby *et al.* 1977). It has been argued that the efficacy of public health interventions may be enhanced with reference to social cognitive models of health behaviour (Conner and Norman 1996; Armitage and Conner 2000). This chapter focuses on Ajzen's (1991) TPB.

2 Theoretical perspective: an extended Theory of Planned Behaviour

2.1 An extended Theory of Planned Behaviour

Ajzen's (1991) TPB posits behavioural intention as the proximal determinant of behaviour. Thus, the more one is motivated (that is, intends) to consume a low-fat diet, for example, the more one is likely actually to do so. Ajzen argues that perceived control is an important codeterminant of behaviour. Generally, the more control one has over a behaviour, the more likely should be its occurrence (cf. Bandura 1997). Typically, perceived control is operationalized in terms of the perceived ease or difficulty of performing a particular behaviour (Sparks *et al.* 1997). Hence, to the extent that individuals accurately perceive control (or a lack of control) over the behaviour, measures of perceived control should independently predict behaviour.

Congruent with recent work, the present study conceptualizes perceived control as consisting of two components (Armitage and Conner 1999a, 1999b): self-efficacy and 'perceived control over behaviour' (see Figure 5.1). The distinction between self-efficacy and perceived control over behaviour is based on distinguishing 'internal' and 'external' influences on level of perceived control. Thus, while eating a low-fat diet may be regarded as being 'difficult', it is possible to delineate internal factors (for example lack of food preparation skills) from external factors (for example availability). Based on work by Bandura (1997), self-efficacy is defined as 'confidence in one's own ability' and relates to feelings of personal competence, ability and skill associated with engaging in the behaviour in question. Perceived control over behaviour (PCB) is concerned with the perceived controllability

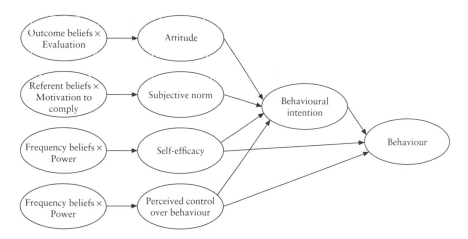

Figure 5.1 Extended Theory of Planned Behaviour

of behaviour, that is, an assessment of environmental constraints on action. Evidence for discriminant validity between self-efficacy and PCB has been found in a number of health settings (for example Dzewaltowski *et al.* 1990; White *et al.* 1994), as well as food choice (for example Armitage and Conner 1999a, 1999b). It should be noted that 'perceived control over behaviour' differs from Ajzen's 'perceived behavioural control' (PCB). The former deliberately excludes measures that ask about the perceived ease or difficulty of performing a particular behaviour.

2.2 Applications of the TPB to food choice

A series of narrative and quantitative reviews have shown the efficacy of the TPB in predicting behaviour in general, and health behaviour in particular (for example Conner and Sparks 1996; Godin and Kok 1996). Further, there have been several applications of the TPB to predict food choice intentions and behaviour, from the use of gene technology in food production (for example Sparks *et al.* 1995) to fat intake (for example Armitage and Conner 1999a, 1999b). For example, Armitage and Conner (1999a) reported that the TPB (extended as here to include self-efficacy and PCB) accounted for 39 per cent of the variance in self-reported consumption of a low-fat diet and 60 per cent of the variance in intention to eat a low-fat diet (see also Sparks *et al.* 1997; Armitage and Conner 1999b).

2.3 Use of the TPB to promote behaviour change

In recent years, relatively little attention has been focused on ways in which the TPB might be used to change behaviour. Indeed, only Fishbein and Ajzen (1975) provide a framework for understanding the way in which models such as the TPB may be used to change behaviour.[2] They emphasize the fact that beliefs are the basic determinants of any behaviour, and that any attempt to change behaviour must therefore be targeted at the underlying beliefs. They argue that successful behavioural change will occur only when intentions are changed through either attitudes or subjective norms. Within the TPB this may also be achieved by changing perceived control (that is, self-efficacy and PCB). The causal model dictates that following (for example) behavioural belief change, attitudes will change and influence behavioural intentions, which will ultimately change behaviour.

Changing behavioural beliefs involves changing individuals' beliefs about the consequences of their actions. More specifically, following a positively valenced persuasive communication, positive outcomes should be seen as more likely to occur, and negative outcomes as less likely to occur. In addition, positive outcomes should be evaluated more positively and negative outcomes more negatively. The normative route would change people's expectations regarding the approval/disapproval of referents, or target their motivation to comply with such referents. Congruent with this, perceived control (that is, self-efficacy and PCB) should increase when facilitating factors are seen as frequent and as exerting a powerful influence over behaviour, and when inhibiting factors are perceived to be infrequent and to exert minimal influence over behaviour.

Fishbein and Ajzen (1975) explicate two strategies by which beliefs may be changed. The first involves introducing new salient beliefs. This approach would expose individuals to new positive salient outcomes associated with the behaviour in question, introduce them to new social referents with whom they were motivated to comply, or introduce new facilitating factors. While the efficacy of this approach remains an empirical question, one attractive feature is that it avoids the extensive piloting required to change existing beliefs. Given that modally salient beliefs provide a good indication of individually salient beliefs (for example Agnew 1998), once the researcher knew the salient beliefs of a small sample of the target group, it would be possible simply to 'brainstorm' novel beliefs. However, there are also significant disadvantages to this approach. First, it seems unlikely that one would be able to generate a list of completely new outcomes when the behaviour is frequently performed (for example 'eating a low-fat diet'). Even if it were possible to develop such an intervention, it would (presumably) be difficult to make such beliefs salient. Indeed, Fishbein and Ajzen provide little indication as to how one would ensure that such beliefs became salient. Second, the approach is somewhat atheoretical, given that one would not be able to evaluate fully the impact of the message. More specifically, without appropriate piloting, it would be impossible to distinguish effects due to belief introduction from (existing) belief change. Fishbein and Ajzen highlight the fact that beliefs may influence a number of other beliefs by inference.

The second strategy focuses on changing existing salient beliefs of the target population. Here, Fishbein and Ajzen (1975) argue that once researchers have identified the salient beliefs of the target population, they can then challenge negative salient beliefs or strengthen positive salient beliefs. Stated thus, however, this approach immediately raises an ambiguity: by definition, government health campaigns focus on (at least) one highly salient outcome of behaviour (that is, health), yet have failed to produce adequate behaviour change. By way of an example, one salient outcome of failing to eat a low-fat diet is the increased risk of heart disease (Armitage and Conner 1999a). Following Fishbein and Ajzen's approach, a persuasive communication might stress the likelihood that eating a low-fat diet would reduce one's risk of heart disease, and that this outcome is positive. However, we would suggest that this would exert very little impact on behaviour. Specifically, Armitage and Conner (1999a: 78) found no difference in either outcome belief or evaluation between those who intended to eat a low-fat diet and those who did not. Thus, both intenders and non-intenders were aware of the link between a low-fat diet and reduced risk of heart disease and evaluated it positively. In this case, an intervention designed to make the link between fat intake and heart disease salient would have little impact, because the belief is already salient, and is in the desired direction.

Changing existing beliefs therefore requires a more fine-grained analysis. In order to develop a TPB-based intervention, the researcher is first required to conduct an empirical study. The study must identify salient beliefs, determine which TPB variables are most predictive of intentions and behaviour, and determine which salient beliefs are likely to prove the most effective targets. This last point is crucial, and focuses on discovering either which beliefs are more predictive of (for example) attitudes, or determining which best discriminate between those who intend to perform the behaviour and those who do not. Although this approach is more intensive and time-consuming than introducing new salient beliefs, it provides a firm basis from which to develop an intervention that is likely to be efficacious and can be usefully evaluated. Moreover, a number of published TPB studies already present such analyses. These provide a framework for other researchers to develop such interventions (for example Armitage and Conner 1999a, 1999b).

There are few direct applications of Fishbein and Ajzen's (1975) principles of behaviour change, although several studies have used the TRA and TPB to plan or evaluate interventions (for example Babrow *et al.* 1990). More directly related to the suggestions of Fishbein and Ajzen (1975), Murphy and Brubaker (1990) designed a video entitled *TSE (Testicular Self-Examination): It can Save your Life* based on the TPB. The video was designed to strengthen and challenge specific outcome beliefs, strengthen perceptions of normative pressure and increase perceptions of control. Exposure to the theory-based message resulted in significantly stronger intentions and actual performance of TSE than occurred in the information or control groups. However, the theoretical intervention was no better than the information-only condition at changing outcome beliefs or attitudes. The latter finding may have been the result of the small sample size (99 participants between 3 groups) and different presentation methods.[3]

More recently, Parker *et al.* (1996) designed four videos aimed at changing normative beliefs, behavioural beliefs, perceived behavioural control, and anticipated regret, with respect to speeding (see also Parker's Chapter 8 in this volume). The normative beliefs and anticipated affect videos had a significant positive impact on attitudes and beliefs, although the perceived behavioural control video decreased perceptions of control, the opposite of what was predicted.

More closely related to the present study, Patterson *et al.* (1996) used social cognitive variables to predict fat, fibre and weight over three years. Although they did not perform any intervention (other than the questionnaire), they found that a strong belief in the diet–cancer relationship and knowledge of National Cancer Institute fat and fibre goals significantly reduced percentage fat intake. Knowledge of both the diet–cancer relationship and the National Cancer Institute goals represent beliefs about specific outcomes. Within the TPB framework, these would be predicted to influence attitudes, intentions and behaviour, respectively. The implication is that the TPB may therefore provide a useful framework for theory-driven dietary interventions (for a review of TPB-based interventions see Hardeman *et al.* 1998).

2.4 Summary

Where the suggestions of Fishbein and Ajzen (1975) have been followed with adequate sample sizes, there has generally been meaningful change in attitudes and other TPB variables. However, it must be noted that there has been little attempt to assess the effect of such interventions on subsequent behaviour. The work we have reviewed has two main implications for our own intervention. First, social cognitive interventions are potentially the safest and most effective way of intervening in dietary behaviour on a large scale,[4] although there has been a dearth of research in this area. Second, data show that the proportion of food energy derived from fat has remained stable since the early 1980s (for example MAFF 1992), in spite of several high-profile health campaigns. Implementation of psychological theory may enhance the modest effects of health promotion to date. Congruent with this, large-scale interventions continue to attract criticism concerning their lack of theoretical grounding (for example Family Heart Study Group 1994; OXCHECK Study Group 1994). The present study was designed to apply Fishbein and Ajzen's (1975) principles of attitude change to influence fat consumption.

3 The intervention

3.1 Design

The study was a randomized controlled trial, designed to assess the efficacy of three dietary interventions, and involved four discrete stages: pilot, baseline, intervention development and implementation, and follow-up. First, modally salient behavioural beliefs were derived from pilot interviews with a representative sample of the target population (n = 20). The interviews were transcribed, and salient behavioural beliefs were identified. These modally salient beliefs informed the content of the TPB questionnaire that was presented at baseline. Following collection of data at baseline, participants were randomly allocated to one of three intervention conditions (information, attitude change, self-efficacy). Intervention materials were distributed three months post-baseline. Changes in TPB variables and dietary intake were assessed at follow-up, five months post-intervention. The attitude change intervention was based on the principles of Fishbein and Ajzen (1975) and was designed to change the salient beliefs that distinguished intenders from non-intenders.

3.2 Participants

A total of 800 people (658 female and 142 male hospital workers) were contacted at baseline (mean age = 36.3 years; range = 17–66 years). Of these, 65 per cent (n = 517) were successfully contacted again at follow-up, eight months later. Data analysis is based upon the 517 individuals (65 per cent of original sample) for whom all data were available. There were 421 females and 96 males, mean age 37.0 years (range = 20–66 years). Responders did not differ from non-responders on any demographic or TPB variables.

3.3 Measures

The measures used were based on our previous research on predicting consumption of a low-fat diet (see Armitage and Conner 1999a, 1999b). All variables were measured using multi-item scales that possessed good internal reliability (that is, Cronbach's alphas of at least 0.70). Fat intake was measured using a validated food frequency questionnaire (see Cade and Margetts 1988; Margetts *et al.* 1989). All measures were taken at both baseline and follow-up.

3.4 Materials

The intervention materials took the form of four-page A5-size leaflets. Two were theory based, the other was designed to provide information only.

Information intervention

This leaflet provided information pertaining to types of fat, UK government recommendations concerning fat intake, and epidemiological data on current UK levels of fat consumption. The information provided in the leaflet formed the basis for the other interventions, which also included theory-based information. In this way it was possible to control for mere presentation of information.

Attitude change intervention

Data from baseline were used to identify the salient beliefs that distinguished those who intended to eat a low-fat diet from those who did not (n = 684; n = 114, respectively). Univariate Fs were used to establish differences in outcome beliefs and outcome evaluations. Differences between behavioural belief products were not considered, due to the difficulty of interpreting multiplicative terms (see Evans 1991).

As predicted, significant differences were found for nearly all outcome beliefs and evaluations (F [10, 769] = 15.65, p < 0.001). In particular, intenders thought that eating a low-fat diet would be more likely to help them stay fit (F [1, 778] = 42.42, p < 0.001), control their weight (F [1, 778] = 44.10, p < 0.001), and make them healthy (F [1, 778] = 51.04, p < 0.001). Intenders generally evaluated these outcomes significantly more posit-ively than non-intenders (F [1, 778] = 4.20, p < 0.05; F [1, 778] = 78.89, p < 0.001; F [1, 778] = 1.84, NS, respectively), although there was no difference between intenders and non-intenders' evaluations of making them feel healthy. In addition, intenders were more unlikely to believe that to become low in fat, foods required too much processing (F [1, 778] = 7.39, p < 0.01), and intenders evaluated this more negatively than non-intenders (F [1, 778] = 6.50, p < 0.05). The value attached to the taste of food did not discriminate between intenders and non-intenders (F [1, 778] = 0.05, NS). This shows that both intenders and non-intenders evaluated tasty food in the same way, while non-intenders believed that food that is low in fat is less likely to taste good (F [1, 778] = 49.46, p < 0.001).

In addition to providing general information, the attitude change inter-vention attempted to target those beliefs that distinguished intenders from non-intenders. That is, positive beliefs held by intenders were strengthened, and negative beliefs refuted. For example, one belief held by non-intenders was that food that is low in fat is less likely to taste good. The attitude intervention made two specific points to counter this: first, that companies producing low-fat foods need to make a profit; and that individuals may simply need to change the preparation method they are currently using in order to lower the fat content of their diet.

Self-efficacy intervention
Ajzen (1991) does not provide specific guidance on how to change beliefs underlying perceptions of control. We therefore followed the suggestions of Bandura (1997). In addition to the standard information, simple, easy-to-follow advice on eating a low-fat diet was provided. For example, the self-efficacy intervention provided recipes for meals that not only were low in fat, but also were cheap, included readily available ingredients, and did not take long to prepare or cook.

3.5 Results

Baseline
MANOVA revealed no differences between conditions on any baseline measures (F [32, 1474] = 1.07, NS). Examination of univariate Fs similarly revealed no between-subjects differences at baseline on demographic and

TPB variables. General intervention effects were assessed using a series of within-subjects MANOVAs, with condition as a between-subjects factor. Dependent variables were TPB components and indicators of fat intake (total, percentage, and saturated).

Intervention effects: TPB variables
Table 5.1 provides data showing the effects of the interventions on TPB variables. There was a significant main effect of time (F [5, 496] = 5.26, p < 0.001), suggesting that the interventions had a significant impact on TPB variables. Contrary to prediction, however, there was no evidence to suggest that the theory-driven interventions were more effective than the knowledge intervention (condition × time interaction: F [10, 992] = 0.69, p = 0.73). In spite of this, univariate tests revealed two significant effects on attitude from the attitude change and self-efficacy enhancement interventions. Both improved attitude towards eating a low-fat diet (t [170] = 3.05, p < 0.001; t [170] = 3.03, p < 0.001, respectively).

Intervention effects: fat intake
Table 5.1 also presents the effects of the interventions on fat intake. Overall, there was a significant main effect of time (F [3, 512] = 9.78, p < 0.001), which was not specifically related to any of the interventions (condition × time interaction: F [6, 1024] = 0.23, p = 0.97). In general, total fat intake and saturated fat intake decreased, while percentage fat intake marginally increased. The attitude and self-efficacy interventions significantly reduced total and saturated fat intake; the knowledge intervention also significantly decreased saturated fat intake. However, mean percentage fat intake was 34.69 per cent (SD = 6.20), indicating that the majority of participants were already eating within the UK government guidelines we had provided for them. We therefore restricted subsequent analysis to individuals consuming *more than* 35 per cent of calories from fat.

Controlling for initial fat intake
We controlled for initial level of fat intake by dividing participants into high- and low-fat consumer groups. High-fat consumers were defined as those currently deriving more than (or equal to) 35 per cent of their calories from fat (n = 417); low-fat consumers were defined as those currently eating less than 35 per cent of calories from fat (n = 383).

Analysis of TPB variables (Table 5.2) revealed that attitude, subjective norm, self-efficacy, PCB and intention differed significantly over time (F [5, 493] = 5.27, p < 0.001), but that such effects were not attributable to either initial fat intake (fat intake × time interaction: F [5, 493] = 1.14, p = 0.34) or condition (condition × time interaction: F [10, 986] = 0.74, p = 0.68). The three-way condition × fat intake × time interaction was similarly non-significant (F [10, 986] = 0.97, p = 0.46).

Table 5.1 Effects of interventions on TPB variables and fat intake

	Information (n = 163)			Attitude (n = 170)			Self-Efficacy (n = 170)		
	Time 1	Time 2	Difference[a]	Time 1	Time 2	Difference[a]	Time 1	Time 2	Difference[a]
TPB variables									
Attitude	1.35 (1.20)	1.41 (1.21)	+0.06	1.16 (1.37)	1.43 (1.26)	+0.27***	1.23 (1.18)	1.46 (1.11)	+0.23***
Subjective norm	4.98 (1.43)	4.96 (1.51)	−0.02	4.84 (1.46)	4.90 (1.34)	+0.06	5.03 (1.41)	4.97 (1.28)	−0.06
Self-efficacy	5.49 (1.29)	5.53 (1.06)	+0.04	5.52 (1.27)	5.50 (1.10)	−0.02	5.47 (1.27)	5.44 (1.31)	−0.03
PCB	5.70 (1.12)	5.57 (1.26)	−0.13	5.82 (1.22)	5.63 (1.28)	−0.14	5.61 (1.30)	5.49 (1.27)	−0.12
Intention	1.56 (1.31)	1.47 (1.39)	−0.09	1.45 (1.53)	1.51 (1.33)	+0.06	1.46 (1.38)	1.37 (1.39)	−0.09
Fat intake									
Total fat (g)	63.22 (27.70)	60.92 (26.19)	−2.30	64.14 (25.56)	61.43 (23.10)	−2.71*	68.08 (30.60)	63.96 (27.91)	−4.12*
Percentage fat	34.27 (6.51)	34.54 (6.66)	+0.27	34.66 (6.10)	35.22 (6.20)	+0.56	35.12 (6.01)	35.49 (6.23)	+0.37
Saturated fat (g)	23.89 (11.53)	22.68 (10.15)	−1.21*	24.28 (10.41)	22.97 (9.17)	−1.31*	25.57 (11.79)	23.85 (11.19)	−1.72*

Notes: [a]Differences in attitudes between Time 1 and Time 2
± signs indicate direction of effect
*p < 0.05   ***p < 0.001

Table 5.2   Effects of interventions by consumer group (difference scores)

	Information (n = 163)		Attitude (n = 170)		Self-Efficacy (n = 170)	
	High Fat[a]	Low Fat[a]	High Fat[a]	Low Fat[a]	High Fat[a]	Low Fat[a]
TPB variables						
Attitude	+0.05	+0.08	+0.34	+0.21	+0.21	+0.26
Subjective norm	−0.30	+0.22	+0.08	+0.03	−0.01	−0.11
Self-efficacy	+0.17	−0.07	−0.01	−0.02	+0.04	−0.11
PCB	−0.03	−0.21	−0.19	−0.18	−0.14	−0.09
Intention	−0.24	+0.03	+0.01	+0.10	−0.08	−0.09
Fat intake						
Total fat (g)	−9.99***	+4.13	−7.48***	+1.79	−8.78***	+0.89
Percentage fat	−1.72***	+1.94	−1.46***	+2.47	−0.95***	+1.86
Saturated fat (g)	−4.54***	+1.60	−3.24***	+0.51	−3.66***	+0.49

Notes: [a]Difference scores between Time 1 and Time 2
± signs indicate direction of effect
***indicate significant (p < 0.001) differences between consumer groups

Analysis of data from the food frequency questionnaire similarly revealed non-significant interactions between condition × fat intake × time (F [6, 1018] = 0.64, p = 0.69) and condition × time (F [6, 1018] = 0.26, p = 0.95). However, there was a significant main effect of time (F [3, 509] = 9.83, p < 0.001) and a significant fat intake × time interaction (F [3, 509] = 20.99, p < 0.001). The latter finding indicates that, while there were no effects attributable to any one of the conditions, there were overall effects that manifested across consumer groups. Thus low-fat consumers tended to consume more fat when faced with the healthy eating material; high-fat consumers significantly reduced their fat intake. Moreover, analysis of the difference scores revealed that this occurred for total, percentage, and saturated fat intake alike (univariate Fs [1, 511] = 28.38, 56.24, 33.36, respectively, all p's < 0.001). This indicates that, while there was no advantage to being in the theoretically driven conditions, there was evidence to suggest that providing these materials to high-fat consumers produced significant change. However, while the proportion of calories derived from fat increased somewhat in low-fat consumers, levels remained within the UK government recommendation of < 35 per cent.

4 Discussion: implications for theory, policy and practice

4.1 Impact of interventions

The present study reported a TPB-based intervention designed to reduce the amount of fat consumed by hospital workers. Across the sample as a whole, there was some evidence to suggest that the theory-driven interventions improved people's attitudes towards eating a low-fat diet, although the effects on fat consumption were limited to total and saturated fat intake. Controlling for initial fat intake, there was evidence to suggest that, while none of the interventions impacted on TPB variables, proportion of fat consumed decreased by more than 1 per cent in high-fat consumers. In low-fat consumers, the dietary interventions *increased* fat intake, but not above government-recommended levels.

While the full generalizability of the intervention is still to be established, a low-intensity dietary intervention could have important public health implications. The technique has the potential to reach large sections of the population. In particular, we managed to reduce percentage of calories derived from fat by more than 1 per cent in high-fat consumers. If one considers that even a 1 per cent reduction in dietary calories derived from fat could result in 10,000 lives saved in the US alone, the present intervention may have an important impact on morbidity and mortality when applied at the population level (see Rose 1985).

4.2 Efficacy of the TPB interventions

Congruent with the findings of Murphy and Brubaker (1990), the TPB-based interventions were no more effective than information only. This may reflect the 'minimalist' nature of the interventions. In attempting to control for the amount of information provided to participants, the information may have minimized differences between conditions. Indeed, as we argued earlier, by definition, any attempt to present individuals with health information represents an attempt to increase the salience of a particular health outcome. Similarly, the Parker *et al.* (1996) study indicated that interventions analogous to the present attitude and self-efficacy interventions had little impact on attitudes or beliefs. The finding that interventions targeting norms and anticipated affect were useful needs to be considered in relation to food choice, particularly considering the role of emotional factors in determining food choice attitudes. Future work is required to test the effects of simultaneously targeting all TPB variables.

4.3 Theoretical implications

Previous research has shown that the TPB typically accounts for 34–58 per cent of the variance in food choice behaviour. The possibility exists that, although this may be impressive in terms of social cognition models (Armitage and Conner 2000), the influence of intention and perceived behavioural control is too small to affect behavioural change. Given that one cannot expect perfect relationships between variables, one might predict only a limited effect on behaviour. In TPB terms, the interventions targeted

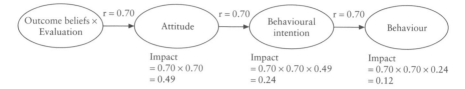

Figure 5.2 Impact of interventions on attitudes and behaviour in the TPB

only distal predictors of behaviour. Figure 5.2 presents a diagrammatic representation of the problem, displaying the proposed causal relationships between beliefs, attitude, behavioural intention and behaviour.[5] Assuming near-perfect correlations between components,[6] one would expect a much weaker effect of any change on behaviour than on attitude. A correlation of 0.70 between behavioural beliefs and attitude means that behavioural beliefs account for 49 per cent of the variance in attitude (that is, $R2 = 0.49$). Assuming a causal relationship between these variables, any impact on attitude is therefore restricted to that 49 per cent of the variance explained by behavioural beliefs. Further assuming that an intervention exerts maximal impact on behavioural beliefs, the level of impact on attitude can be expressed as the proportion of variance explained in attitude (that is, $0.70 \times 0.70 = 0.49$). As Figure 5.2 shows, the impact of the intervention will diminish as one moves further down the causal chain. The implication is that, even under ideal conditions, one might expect only modest effects on behaviour, although at the level of public health this might be of considerable practical use (cf. Rose 1985).

One alternative strategy might therefore usefully focus on investigating ways in which the more proximal determinants of behaviour may be influenced directly. For example, there may be variables other than beliefs that influence attitude, subjective norm, self-efficacy and PCB. Recent work on breast self-examination and vitamin supplement taking, for example, has shown that encouraging people to make plans about when and where they will implement their intentions has a significant impact on people's behaviour (see Orbell *et al.* 1997; Sheeran and Orbell 1999; Orbell and Sheeran, Chapter 7 in this volume). Congruent with this, the interventions that do have an impact on behaviour tend to be intensive, either mass communication or one-to-one counselling (for example Maccoby *et al.* 1977).

4.4 Limitations

In this study, there were a number of problems associated with the leaflet medium. First, there was no control over whether participants read their leaflets. Second, it is possible that participants may have seen more than one theory-based intervention. Third, several studies (for example Maccoby *et al.* 1977) have shown the usefulness of alternative media for intervening in dietary behaviour. The findings therefore echo those of Chaiken and Eagly (1983), who reported that videos were more effective than either audio or written messages, and that of these, the written medium was least effective in changing attitudes (cf. Parker *et al.* 1996). While the approach might be less costly, it is also less effective. Additional comparison groups would deal with these limitations.

4.5 Future directions

Recent work in the field of public health has shown that tailoring messages enhances the effectiveness of persuasive communications. For example, Brug *et al.*'s (1996) study targeted the beliefs of individuals (as opposed to 'intenders' or 'non-intenders'), and significantly reduced fat consumption. Thus, one possibility for future research would be to use a more fine-grained analysis to target interventions more carefully. However, while this approach may exert greater influence on behaviour, it would also move health promotion attempts towards more intensive intervention.

Related to this discussion, it has been suggested that the use of modally salient beliefs in the TPB may be too general to tap individual concerns. Given that these formed the basis of our attitude change intervention, it is possible that the targeted beliefs were too general. However, studies examining the relative merits of providing individually derived beliefs from modally salient beliefs have generally found little added benefit (for example Agnew 1998). Indeed, Agnew (1998: 271) concludes that 'practical considerations may outweigh the modest gain in predictive accuracy'. A related approach might be to target the beliefs that are regarded as being important. For example, Van der Pligt and de Vries (1998) provide evidence to suggest that important beliefs are more predictive. While the authors acknowledge the difficulties associated with distinguishing between salience and importance, it seems likely that while all important beliefs are likely to be salient, not all salient beliefs will be regarded as important. Hence, future studies might target individuals' most important beliefs.

The present study provided little evidence to support a role for the TPB in changing food choice behaviour. However, given the limitations outlined above, it is clear that alternative applications of the model may influence behaviour change. In particular, further experimentation with alternative intervention media and further integration with work on tailoring and planning may produce greater behaviour change.

Acknowledgement

The authors would like to thank Dr Paul Sparks for his valuable comments on an earlier draft of this chapter.

Notes

1 Note that these are UK government recommendations, and may be regarded as being relatively 'lenient'. In the USA, for example, government recommendations are considerably lower than those for the UK: 30 per cent of food energy from fat (US Department of Health and Human Services 1991).
2 Note that Fishbein and Ajzen's (1975) discussion focuses on the Theory of Reasoned Action, an earlier version of the TPB which does not include measures of perceived control (that is, self-efficacy and PCB).
3 The experimental group received a video; information received audio tape and slides; control was a leaflet.
4 See Jacobs (1993) and Temple (1996) for a discussion of increased mortality associated with pharmacological interventions.
5 For simplicity, this discussion focuses on attitudes, but for the most part, a similar pattern would be expected for subjective norms, self-efficacy and PCB. Note, however, that one might expect changes in self-efficacy and PCB to bypass intentions and influence behaviour directly (Figure 5.1).
6 Note that any correlation greater than 0.70 would imply a lack of discriminant validity between components, introducing problems of multicollinearity (see Tabachnick and Fidell 1989).

References

Agnew, C.R. (1998) Modal versus individually-derived beliefs about condom use: measuring the cognitive underpinnings of the theory of reasoned action, *Psychology and Health*, 13: 271–87.
Ajzen, I. (1991) The Theory of Planned Behavior, *Organizational Behavior and Human Decision Processes*, 50: 179–211.
Armitage, C.J. and Conner, M. (1999a) Distinguishing perceptions of control from self-efficacy: predicting consumption of a low fat diet using the theory of planned behavior, *Journal of Applied Social Psychology*, 29: 72–90.
Armitage, C.J. and Conner, M. (1999b) The theory of planned behaviour: assessment of predictive validity and 'perceived control', *British Journal of Social Psychology*, 38: 35–54.
Armitage, C.J. and Conner, M. (2000) Social cognition models and health behaviour: a structured review, *Psychology and Health*, 15: 173–89.
Babrow, A.S., Black, D.R. and Tiffany, S.T. (1990) Beliefs, attitudes, intentions, and a smoking-cessation program: a planned behavior analysis of communication campaign development, *Health Communication*, 2(3): 145–63.
Bandura, A. (1997) *Self-Efficacy: The Exercise of Control*. New York: Freeman.
Brug, J., Steenhuis, I., van Assema, P. and de Vries, H. (1996) The impact of a computer-tailored nutrition intervention, *Preventive Medicine*, 25: 236–42.
Cade, J.E. and Margetts, B.M. (1988) Nutrient sources in the English diet: quantitative data from three English towns, *International Journal of Epidemiology*, 17: 844–8.

Chaiken, S. and Eagly, A.H. (1983) Communication modality as a determinant of persuasion: the role of communicator salience, *Journal of Personality and Social Psychology*, 45: 241–56.

Conner, M. and Norman, P. (eds) (1996) *Predicting Health Behaviour: Research and Practice with Social Cognition Models*. Buckingham: Open University Press.

Conner, M. and Sparks, P. (1996) The theory of planned behaviour and health behaviours, in M. Conner and P. Norman (eds) *Predicting Health Behaviour: Research and Practice with Social Cognition Models*. Buckingham: Open University Press.

Department of Health (1992) *The Health of the Nation: A Strategy for Health in England*. London: HMSO.

Dzewaltowski, D.A., Noble, J.M. and Shaw, J.M. (1990) Physical activity participation: social cognitive theory versus the theories of reasoned action and planned behavior, *Journal of Sport and Exercise Psychology*, 12: 388–405.

Evans, M.G. (1991) The problem of analyzing multiplicative composites: interactions revisited, *American Psychologist*, 46(1): 6–15.

Family Heart Study Group (1994) Randomised controlled trial evaluating cardiovascular screening and intervention in general practice: principal results of the British Family Heart Study, *British Medical Journal*, 308: 313–20.

Fishbein, M. and Ajzen, I. (1975) *Belief, Attitude, Intention and Behavior: An Introduction to Theory and Research*. Reading, MA: Addison-Wesley.

Godin, G. and Kok, G. (1996) The Theory of Planned Behavior: a review of its applications to health-related behaviors, *American Journal of Health Promotion*, 11(2): 87–98.

Hardeman, W., Johnston, M., Kinmonth, A.L. and Wareham, N. (1998) The use of the theory of planned behaviour in interventions: a systematic review. Poster presented at the British Psychological Society's Division of Health Psychology annual conference, University of Wales Bangor, UK, July.

Jacobs, D.R., Jr (1993) Why is low blood cholesterol associated with risk of nonatherosclerotic disease death?, *Annual Review of Public Health*, 14: 95–114.

Maccoby, N., Farquhar, J.W., Wood, P.D. and Alexander, J. (1977) Reducing the risk of cardiovascular disease: effects of a community-based campaign on knowledge and behavior, *Journal of Community Health*, 3: 100–14.

Margetts, B.M., Cade, J.E. and Osmond, C. (1989) Comparison of a food frequency questionnaire with a diet record, *International Journal of Epidemiology*, 18: 868–73.

Ministry of Agriculture, Fisheries and Food (MAFF) (1992) *Manual of Nutrition*. London: HMSO.

Murphy, W.G. and Brubaker, R.G. (1990) Effects of a brief theory-based intervention on the practice of testicular self-examination by high school males, *Journal of School Health*, 60: 459–62.

Oomura, Y., Tarui, S., Inoue, S. and Shimazu, T. (eds) (1991) *Progress in Obesity Research*. London: John Libbey.

Orbell, S., Hodgkins, S. and Sheeran, P. (1997) Implementation intentions and the theory of planned behavior, *Personality and Social Psychology Bulletin*, 23(9): 945–54.

OXCHECK Study Group (1994) Effectiveness of health checks conducted by nurses in primary care: results of the OXCHECK study after one year, *British Medical Journal*, 308: 308–12.

Parker, D., Stradling, S.G. and Manstead, A.S.R. (1996) Modifying beliefs and attitudes to exceeding the speed limit: an intervention study based on the theory of planned behavior, *Journal of Applied Social Psychology*, 26(1): 1–19.

Patterson, R.E., Kristal, A.R. and White, E. (1996) Do beliefs, knowledge, and perceived norms about diet and cancer predict dietary change?, *American Journal of Public Health*, 86: 1394–400.

Rose, G. (1985) Sick individuals and sick populations, *International Journal of Epidemiology*, 14: 32–8.

Schapira, D.V., Kumar, N.B., Lyman, G.H. and Baile, W.F. (1991) The effect of duration of intervention and locus of control on dietary change, *American Journal of Preventive Medicine*, 7: 341–7.

Sheeran, P. and Orbell, S. (1999) Implementation intentions and repeated behaviour: augmenting the predictive validity of the theory of planned behaviour, *European Journal of Social Psychology*, 29: 349–69.

Sparks, P., Shepherd, R. and Frewer, L.J. (1995) Assessing and structuring attitudes toward the use of gene technology in food production: the role of perceived ethical obligation, *Basic and Applied Social Psychology*, 16: 267–85.

Sparks, P., Guthrie, C.A. and Shepherd, R. (1997) The dimensional structure of the perceived behavioral control construct, *Journal of Applied Social Psychology*, 27(5): 418–38.

Stallones, R.A. (1983) Ischemic heart disease and lipids in blood and diet, *Annual Review of Nutrition*, 3: 155–85.

Tabachnick, B.G. and Fidell, L.S. (1989) *Using Multivariate Statistics*. New York: HarperCollins.

Temple, N.J. (1996) Dietary fats and coronary heart disease, *Biomedicine and Pharmacotherapy*, 50: 261–8.

Trichopoulos, D. and Willett, D.C. (eds) (1996) Nutrition and cancer [special issue], *Cancer Causes and Control*, 7(1).

US Department of Health and Human Services (1991) *Healthy People 2000: National Health Promotion and Disease Prevention Objectives*. Washington, DC: US Department of Health and Human Services.

Van der Pligt, J. and de Vries, N.K. (1998) Belief importance in expectancy-value models of attitudes, *Journal of Applied Social Psychology*, 28: 1339–54.

Westerterp, K.R., Verboeket-van de Venne, W.P.H.G., Westerterp-Plantenga, M.S. *et al.* (1996) Dietary and body fat: an intervention study, *International Journal of Obesity*, 20: 1022–6.

White, K.M., Terry, D. and Hogg, M.A. (1994) Safer sex behavior: the role of attitudes, norms, and control factors, *Journal of Applied Social Psychology*, 24(24): 2164–92.

6

SARA WILLIAMSON AND
JANE WARDLE

INCREASING PARTICIPATION WITH COLORECTAL CANCER SCREENING: THE DEVELOPMENT OF A PSYCHO-EDUCATIONAL INTERVENTION

This chapter describes the development and delivery of a psycho-educational intervention to increase uptake of a new bowel cancer screening test. In order to be effective, the intervention not only had to tackle the barriers associated with any screening programme (for example fear of negative outcome, lack of perceived risk), but also had to identify and reduce barriers specific to this test. One potential barrier is lack of familiarity, as this type of test has never been used before as a screening method in the general UK population, and bowel cancer has received relatively little publicity. As a result, knowledge and awareness of the severity and risk of bowel cancer and thus of need for screening may be expected to be low among the general public. Second, the screening procedure is invasive and could be viewed as embarrassing and painful. In addition, the way in which the test was delivered required participants to volunteer to attend for screening as opposed to complying with a doctor's request. A theoretical approach to the intervention was taken. Rather than presenting factual medical/procedural information, the intervention materials were designed to take the potential participant through the screening decision, addressing the potential barriers and highlighting the benefits. Preliminary results show that the intervention had positive effects on participants' attitudes, beliefs, and intention to attend.

1 Increasing participation with colorectal cancer screening

1.1 What is known about colorectal cancer and what screening methods are available?

Colorectal cancer (often known as bowel cancer) is the second most common cause of cancer death in the UK (Office for National Statistics 1998). The five-year survival rate is relatively poor (37 per cent), principally because, in the majority of cases, the disease has already reached an advanced stage at the point of diagnosis (Austoker 1994). If it is detected at the asymptomatic, localized stage, survival rates are much higher, at around 82–7 per cent (Hart *et al.* 1995). There is a well-established premalignant stage (adenomatous polyps). The estimated time for progression from adenomatous bowel polyps to carcinoma (cancer) is between 10 and 35 years (Austoker 1994). Detecting and removing the polyps should prevent a substantial proportion of bowel cancers. The best hopes for a reduction in bowel cancer mortality in the near future lie in the use of screening methods to detect the disease at a premalignant or early stage.

The two main methods available for population screening for bowel cancer are faecal occult blood testing (FOBT) and sigmoidoscopy. FOBT involves examining the stool for the presence of occult blood. Population screening with the technique offers the prospect of a 15 per cent decrease in mortality (Hardcastle *et al.* 1996; Kronberg *et al.* 1996), through diagnosing cancer at an early pathological stage. FOBT is comparatively inexpensive, but one major disadvantage is its low sensitivity: about 40 per cent of cancers and 80 per cent of adenomas are missed by the test. It also has low specificity, a high rate of false positive results entailing unnecessary follow-up. Sigmoidoscopy is a more expensive and invasive initial test, which involves the insertion of a sigmoidoscope into the bowel to search for polyps and cancers. It is highly sensitive for polyps as small as 5mm, and neoplasia (cell change) is thus detectable at a very early stage. Second, polyps can be removed endoscopically at the time of screening in most cases, which means that the procedure is both diagnostic and therapeutic. Case control studies indicate that screening using flexible sigmoidoscopy (FS) may substantially reduce mortality from colorectal cancers (Newcomb *et al.* 1992; Selby *et al.* 1992) but, until a randomized controlled trial has been undertaken, its efficacy remains unproven. A multi-centre, randomized controlled trial of FS is currently under way in the UK to determine the effect of once-only FS screening on bowel cancer morbidity and mortality. More than 90 per cent of colorectal cancers are diagnosed after 55 years of age, and the prevalence of distal adenomas also increases strikingly after 50 but reaches a plateau at about 60 (Atkin *et al.* 1993). A single sigmoidoscopy performed between the ages of 55 and 64 should therefore identify most people with distal adenomas that are likely to develop into cancers.

1.2 Compliance with bowel cancer screening

In the 1992 and 1993 Behavioural Risk Factor Surveillance System surveys, fewer than 30 per cent of American adults aged 50 and over reported having an FOBT in the past year, or a sigmoidoscopy in the previous five years, despite the tests being widely publicized by the American Cancer Society (1996) and National Cancer Institute (Centers for Disease Control (CDC) 1996). Similar levels of compliance have been found (20–50 per cent) when FOBT has been offered in primary care and community settings in the USA, Australia and Europe (Farrands *et al.* 1984; Macrae *et al.* 1984; Myers *et al.* 1991; Mant *et al.* 1992; Hyman *et al.* 1994; Herbert *et al.* 1997).

There are fewer studies of compliance with sigmoidoscopy. An Australian study used a database from the Electoral Commission to mail invitations to 3500 adults aged 50–59. Fewer than 10 per cent consented to the test (Olynyk *et al.* 1996). However, another Australian study found that when the test was recommended by general practitioners (GPs) during a routine consultation, the attendance rate among 187 older adults was 49 per cent (Cockburn *et al.* 1995). Attendance at the first two screening centres in the UK FS Trial was very high (71 per cent), although this was among individuals who had previously expressed an interest in FS screening (79 per cent).

1.3 Determinants of participation in bowel cancer screening

In order to maximize compliance it is important to understand the determinants of participation in screening. Examples of the more general determinants include the cost of the test, its availability and accessibility, and the publicity about it. Individuals need to know that the test exists, who it is aimed at (for example high-risk groups, specific age groups), where it is available, and whether it is offered free of charge. They also need procedural information, such as how to arrange an appointment.

The two main demographic factors usually associated with higher screening compliance are higher income and education (Brown *et al.* 1990; Neilson and Whynes 1995; CDC 1996). Gender effects have also been noted – men have been found to have higher rates of participation than women (Cockburn *et al.* 1995; Elwood 1997; Herbert *et al.* 1997) – and there are age effects too, though they are not consistent (Macrae *et al.* 1986; Blalock *et al.* 1987; Myers *et al.* 1994; Weller *et al.* 1995).

Family history of bowel cancer (Morrow and Morrell 1982; Macrae *et al.* 1984, 1986; Weller *et al.* 1995) and the presence of bowel symptoms (Macrae *et al.* 1984) have also been associated with higher levels of participation, suggesting a possible link with perceived risk of the disease. Studies of compliance with FOBT reveal that the most common reported reasons for *non-participation* are lack of awareness of the prevalence of bowel cancer, the perceived unpleasantness of the test, absence of bowel symptoms, and fear of further investigations or surgery (Spector *et al.* 1981; Farrands *et al.* 1984; Klaaborg *et al.* 1986; Arveux *et al.* 1992; Hynam *et al.* 1995; Hart *et al.* 1997). Vernon (1997) summarized the findings on non-participation with flexible sigmoidoscopy and indicated that the four reasons most frequently endorsed were very similar to those for FOBT: absence of current health problems or symptoms; practical reasons, such as time and travel constraints; worries about pain; and not wanting to know about health problems.

As a preliminary to our own FS trial, the determinants of interest in bowel cancer screening were examined in a population survey of adults aged 55–64. Participants were asked 'If you were invited to have the bowel cancer screening test, would you take up the offer?' The main predictors of likely uptake were being male, being married or cohabiting, and being employed; having a positive family history, more bowel symptoms, and a previous history of bowel disease; having a higher perceived risk of bowel cancer and worrying more about it; and *not* regarding the test as embarrassing, uncomfortable, time consuming, worrying or tempting fate (Wardle *et al.* 2000).

1.4 Previous interventions

A number of interventions aimed at increasing attendance at cancer screening have been developed and tested already. Byles *et al.* (1995) tested two direct mail strategies (information letter vs information letter, pamphlet and prompt cards) designed to encourage women to have cervical smears. Both interventions resulted in significant increases in attendance, but there were no differences between the two forms of information. For colorectal cancer screening, Thompson *et al.* (1986) tested several 'clinically feasible' strategies that primary care physicians could use routinely to increase participation in FOB testing. They included physician/nurse talk, postcard reminder and telephone reminder. All three strategies produced greater compliance than in the control group, and the postcard reminder was the most effective.

Another possible method at the population level is to use health education leaflets. There is evidence both for and against their effectiveness in increasing participation in colorectal cancer screening. Hardcastle *et al.* (1983) found that by sending an educational letter two weeks before inviting people for FOB screening, compliance was increased by approximately 9 per cent. Hart *et al.* (1997) found that health education leaflets that contained information on screening and also addressed compliance (for example the test is of help to people who may feel well and have no symptoms) increased attendance significantly in men, but not in women. They gave two possible explanations: that men may be less aware of the concept of asymptomatic illness and the benefits of early detection because there are no national screening programmes for men in the UK, and so may be more influenced by the leaflet; and that women may be less persuaded by the leaflet because of previous unpleasant screening experiences.

Not all outcomes of health education interventions have been so positive. Pye *et al.* (1988), for example, found that their health education leaflet *decreased* FOBT compliance by 9 per cent when it was accompanied by a doctor's letter. They suggested that the feeling of a personal invitation was removed by the educational leaflet and that the possibility of individual benefit seemed so small as to make the ordeal of investigation unattractive. The fear-arousing style of the information may also have played a part. The first paragraph, for example, indicated that most people seek help too late, by which time a major operation will be needed and only one in four people will be cured. Nichols *et al.* (1986) compared several methods and found that an educational leaflet about bowel disorder and screening for bowel cancer and polyps had no effect on compliance. They offered no explanation, but the method they found most effective was to make screening available during routine GP consultations. Although the various results are inconsistent, it would appear in summary that information presented in a personal and acceptable format can increase attendance for screening. When designing an intervention it is essential to begin with good data on the predictors of participation in the relevant population, and then to collect detailed data on the proximal effect of the intervention to test whether it impacts on the intended cognitive or emotional processes. Finally, large-scale, randomized control data on attendance are needed, to provide robust estimates of the effect of the intervention.

2 Theoretical perspective: the expectancy value models

2.1 Theoretical models influencing the design and content of the intervention

Our quantitative studies of the determinants of FS screening were designed within the framework of the Health Belief Model (Becker 1974). In the qualitative studies, additional concepts from other theoretical models were utilized, including anticipated affective responses, self-efficacy and social norms.

2.2 Who should be the target for the intervention?

Potential participants received an initial questionnaire to determine their interest in attending for screening. In the first two screening centres that we approached, 57 per cent of respondents expressed 'definite interest', 22 per cent expressed 'probable interest', 12 per cent were 'probably not interested' and 10 per cent were 'definitely not interested'. Only those expressing definite or probable interest were invited for screening. Overall attendance was 71 per cent: 79 per cent among participants expressing definite interest, but only 50 per cent among those expressing probable interest. The 'probably interested' participants perceived more barriers and fewer benefits to screening than the 'definitely interested' and were therefore chosen as our target group. The remainder of the chapter describes the development of the intervention and preliminary data on its impact on attitudes, expectations, and intentions to attend.

2.3 What should be the target of the intervention?

The FS trial gave us the opportunity to study factors associated with screening interest and attendance using data collected before the invitations had been sent out (see Wardle *et al.* 2000 for a full discussion of the predictors of screening interest). From these data we identified the more modifiable determinants of screening and devised a theoretically based intervention aimed at addressing those factors. The intervention had to be inexpensive to produce and disseminate, so a booklet format was adopted. The main aims of the booklet were to promote positive attitudes towards FS screening, to reduce anxiety about screening, to reduce negative expectations and to raise social norms for participation and thereby increase attendance.

3 The intervention

As part of the FS trial, quantitative data were collected from participants at various stages in the screening process in all centres. Existing data from the first two centres (Welwyn Garden City and Leicester) were analysed, and telephone interviews were carried out to examine particular issues in more detail and to clarify points raised in the quantitative analyses. The aims of the analyses were to explore the determinants of screening participation, to identify the modifiable factors that predict interest in the FS test and participation in screening, and to identify the main barriers to screening.

3.1 Quantitative questionnaire study

Baseline data from questionnaires sent out to potential trial participants revealed several factors associated with interest. One was reported worry about bowel cancer: those participants who were 'quite worried' were the most interested; those who were 'not at all worried' or 'very worried' were the least interested. Perceived risk of bowel cancer, personal and family history of bowel disease, reported bowel symptoms, perceived benefits and fewer perceived barriers, and positive attitudes to medical testing were all associated with screening interest.

As screening interest was measured on a four-point scale, it was possible to compare the 'definitely interested' group with the 'probably interested' group to determine which of the attitude and belief measures were the most important. The items where the differences were greatest included: 'The test would take up too much time', 'The test may make me worry about cancer', 'The test would be embarrassing', 'The test would be tempting fate' and 'The test would give me peace of mind.' The 'probably interested' group were more likely to agree with the negative statements and less likely to agree with the positive statements.

3.2 Qualitative studies

Interview data

Interviews were conducted with Leicester trial participants (n = 80; including people who were screened, participants not interested in the test, and non-responders) to highlight and examine important issues that could be addressed by the intervention booklet. Issues examined included reasons for response, reasons for interest/non-interest, barriers to the test, experience of trial, time perspective, anticipated affective response, and normative beliefs.

For *reasons for response/interest in the FS test*, the most common theme to emerge was 'It's better to prevent than treat.' Others included concerns about health, family history of cancer, to gain reassurance, being recommended to go by others, knowing of people who have had cancer/polyps, and to help cancer research.

The most important *barriers* to emerge were these:

- Perceived insusceptibility: the feeling that screening is not necessary because the participant has no symptoms and feels healthy. Family history was also mentioned, sometimes as a prompt to go for screening, sometimes because it increased the respondent's fears and resulted in avoidance of screening.
- Efficacy: some individuals stated that they did not understand what screening was about, and others felt that they did not know what to expect. Both were given as reasons not to go for screening.
- Going for the test may cause problems/cancer.
- Travel: distance to the hospital or the difficulty of the journey.
- Lack of support: having no one to go with to the screening centre or to offer care after the test.
- Fatalistic attitudes: 'Leave well alone – what you don't know can't hurt you', 'What will be will be', 'If I've got it, it's best not to know' and 'We've all got cancer in us.'

- Avoid thinking about the future: the majority of interviewees were 'present focused', concentrating on the 'here and now', and appeared not to want to worry or think about the future.

The anticipated *experience of the test* was a further barrier for some. The majority felt anxious and apprehensive before the test, a small but significant proportion extremely so. A couple of interviewees even reported having second thoughts about whether to go through with the test. However, those who received a 'clear' result, or had polyps but no evidence of cancer, reported that they felt relieved and pleased after the test.

As for *normative beliefs*, the most important referents included partners and children, friends, other family members, and health workers. These were seen as people with whom to discuss the test and make the decision about attending. A few interviewees highlighted the importance of GPs. Those who were interested in having the test were more likely to have discussed it with someone than those who were not interested. Most interviewees thought that people like them would have similar views and would make similar decisions. Several said that individuals with symptoms would be more likely to want the test and should be more concerned about taking up the invitation. The majority felt that others should go for the test, but that it should be the individual's decision. Knowing what other people had decided to do made no difference to the individual's own decision.

Finally, *time perspective* appeared to have little significance for the majority of respondents. A few said that, when making their decision, they had anticipated how they might feel if they had the test. Those who were interested said that the opportunity to prevent cancer was an important consideration, along with anticipated relief, while those who were not interested in having the test mentioned the fear of discovering something wrong as an influential factor.

Questionnaire comments

To examine the test's acceptability, people who were screened were given a short questionnaire the day after the test. A space was provided for comments, and the majority were extremely positive – most frequently thanking the staff for their kindness. A number of useful themes emerged. Embarrassment was raised many times, but respondents consistently reported being far less embarrassed than they had expected. Having confidence in the hospital staff was often mentioned too. Ways of coping with the test were also highlighted: watching the test on the monitor, or talking to the nurse to take the mind off discomfort. The time taken for the test came up many times: 'It really was as quick as had been suggested.' As to the procedure, many people said that the test was nothing to get upset about, and that the thought was worse than the test itself. Normative beliefs were also highlighted: for example, one person said 'Besides reassuring oneself, it also gives greater confidence to fellow family members.'

3.3 The intervention booklet

The purpose of the booklet that we went on to design was to reduce perceived barriers to the test and increase positive beliefs and attitudes in an attempt to improve uptake among participants who were only 'probably interested' in attending. The quantitative and qualitative data we had collected provided a useful basis on which to build the intervention. It was decided that the booklet should contain no additional information concerning the test, beyond that already provided. Rather, it was designed to tackle important psychological barriers to screening, using data from trial participants' personal experiences of the test. The booklet acknowledges potential barriers, suggests possible coping strategies, and presents alternative views. It provides readers with a rehearsal of the benefits of FS screening and directs their attention to the positive emotional impact of screening. It also provides normative information, and models ways of seeking social support.

Presenting effective health education messages is a complex process, because its aim is usually to influence attitudes or behaviour, and not merely to present information (Charlton 1986). Research suggests that much of the available health education literature requires a level of reading ability that makes it inaccessible to those in greatest need of health information (Michielutte *et al.* 1992). Michielutte *et al.* argue that aids such as illustrations and clear text style should be used to make health education literature more accessible to less educated people, while retaining sufficient interest for all reading abilities.

Our FS screening booklet was professionally drawn and set out. The content is clear, direct and personal, and the text is well spaced and printed in easy-to-read typefaces. The booklet adopts a coping rather than mastery approach, in that barriers are acknowledged and solutions proposed, rather than ignored or denied. Vahabi and Ferris (1995) suggested that a conversational narrative style, consisting of short paragraphs, can stimulate and motivate people to read the entire message. Questions and answers about screening are therefore presented in the form of brief conversations between friends and family. Each conversation tackles a particular barrier and is followed by a summary paragraph. Humour is also used, in the form of cartoons, to make the topic more approachable. Quotations from participants screened already are included to give credibility. The booklet is introduced as designed 'for people in your age group, based on surveys with people who have been invited'.

The booklet has three main sections. The first is an information page that repeats material given to participants already about the FS test: the importance of screening, the effectiveness of the test, and information on the likely outcome. The second is a series of cartoons that follow two characters (Mr and Mrs Jones) through the decision to attend screening or not. Seven barriers are identified: fear of discomfort, fear of cancer, fear of embarrassment, concern that the test is not necessary, dislike of medical tests, the idea that it is better to 'leave well alone', and the time taken for the test. Each barrier is identified, possible solutions are offered, and a professional comment is given. The role of social support in health behaviour decisions is also addressed in the form of a cartoon encouraging participants to ask someone to accompany them to the test. Several cartoons show Mr and Mrs Jones talking to others, to emphasize the 'normality' of testing. The cartoon section adopts a conversational style, in which the two characters are seen interacting with important others, such as their family, their friends, their GP and the Flexi-Scope trial administrator. It is hoped that the cartoons will encourage readers to anticipate what the important people in their lives would want them to do and will encourage them to discuss the test with them. The final section of the booklet utilizes anticipated affective response theories, and encourages readers to think about the positive feelings they may experience after the test. Quotations from trial participants are reproduced to demonstrate each point.

3.4 Evaluation study on the intervention booklet

The booklet was piloted with several groups of people involved in the FS trial, and its readability was tested using the Flesch readability formula, which calculates reading ease from a document's average word length and sentence length. It is recommended that readability for the general population should be between 60 and 70 (Vahabi and Ferris 1995), where 100 indicates that the text is very easy to read. The booklet scores 71.

The pilot research was designed to gain feedback from people who were considering having the test and from others who had had it already. Both qualitative (interview) and quantitative (questionnaire) data were collected. The booklet and a semi-structured questionnaire were sent to 50 recently screened participants, with an accompanying letter asking for their assistance; 31 responded. The focus of the quantitative research was how effectively the booklet deals with the common barriers to screening, and whether it has the potential to allay fears and concerns about the test; 100 participants (50 recently screened and 50 who had been invited) were sent the booklet with an accompanying letter inviting them to take part in a telephone interview. Of these, 58 accepted: 2 others refused, and the remainder were unobtainable. The interviews were semi-structured and lasted 5–10 minutes.

The *questionnaire data* revealed that the overall impression of the booklet was positive: the majority of respondents found it very useful (58 per cent), informative (84 per cent reported that it provided all/most of the information they wanted) and very easy to understand (97 per cent). The booklet was seen as effective in dealing with the concerns and worries that people had experienced before the test, but a number of suggestions were made as to how it could be improved: for example, more information about how the bowel is prepared, and other details of procedure; and more facts on how often people should be tested and who is most at risk. Taken together, the results indicate that the booklet was effective in reducing concerns about the FS test, was useful, and was well received. The understandable wish for more information was noted, but space limitations constrained how much material could be included.

The *interviews with screened participants* showed similarly that the booklet was well received: informative, relevant, pertinent and easy to understand. The most frequent criticism was about the illustrations and the humorous approach that had been adopted. The majority of respondents, however, were positive about this aspect of what they saw, and those who were critical nevertheless recognized the value of humour. Our conclusion was to tone down the humour but not to abandon it.

The *interviews with participants who had been invited for the test but not yet tested* revealed positive responses once again. The booklet had made a significant impact on respondents' decisions to have the test, and was said to be informative, reassuring and easy to understand. The cartoons this time were well received. Two additional types of information were said to be missing, however: the procedures used during the test, and how the bowel was prepared. Nevertheless, no amendments were made, since both types of information were provided through other information sheets at the appropriate time.

To take account of what we regarded as the most important points from the feedback, we made a number of changes to the booklet before the full intervention began. The main ones were to modify the cover and to make the illustrations smaller and less prominent. The request for further information about how the bowel was prepared was dealt with through separate information sheets. No changes were made to the information included about the test procedures themselves.

3.5 The intervention study

The intervention study has taken place in seven trial centres. Participants who responded 'Yes probably' to the screening interest question ('If you were invited to have the bowel cancer screening test, would you take up the offer?') were randomized to one of two groups – Booklet/No booklet. Uptake among 'probably interested' participants usually ranges from 35 to 55 per cent, so there is considerable scope for improvement. The impact of the booklet has been assessed initially with a questionnaire on attitudes, expectations and intention sent out with the booklet or at the equivalent time for controls. Attendance will be recorded in due course, after screening invitations have been sent out.

A total of 2966 participants who had indicated that they would only 'probably' attend were identified across the seven centres. In cases where a couple from the same household had been invited, both were sent a copy of the booklet if one had expressed probable interest and the other definite interest; 1453 participants (49 per cent) were allocated to the intervention condition and 1513 (51 per cent) to the control condition. Both groups received a letter with the questionnaire asking them to complete and return it. Those who received a booklet and a questionnaire were encouraged to read the booklet before completing the questionnaire.

Measures

The questionnaire measured a large number of variables, the first of them *demographic*. Age and gender were known from the Family Health Services Authority registers, but there were simple questions about ethnicity (white; black; Asian; other; do not wish to answer), occupational status (working full-time; part-time; not working at present; retired), access to a car (yes; no), educational qualifications (School Certificate; GCE O Level, and so on); housing tenure (owning; renting), and marital status (married or living as married; divorced; separated; widowed; single). *Subjective health* was assessed with a single item ('Would you say that for someone of your age, your health in general is excellent/good/fair/poor?'). Seven bowel symptoms were listed (constipation, diarrhoea, wind, pain, incontinence, blood and haemorrhoids), and participants were asked to rate each one for frequency in the past three months (never, occasionally, frequently). *Perceived risk* and *worry about bowel cancer* were assessed with single questions. The risk item was based on the standard format for assessing optimistic bias, and asked respondents if they felt that their chances of developing bowel cancer were 'lower than', 'about the same as' or 'higher than' those of other men or women of their age. The worry item asked respondents if they were 'not worried at all', 'a bit worried', 'quite worried' or 'very worried' about bowel cancer.

In addition to the above items, a number of statements were presented about cancer and FS screening. In each case, respondents were asked to check one of five response options ('Strongly disagree', 'Disagree', 'Not sure', 'Agree', 'Strongly agree'). The items were entered into a factor analysis and two factors emerged. The first was *positive screening attitudes*: 'Test would be reassuring', 'I would make time for the test', 'Make you feel that you were doing something positive about your health', 'Ought to take the opportunity', 'If I don't go, I might later wish I'd been tested', 'People ought to make the effort to go' and 'Test is important' (Cronbach's alpha = 0.83). The second factor, *discomfort*, comprised 'Embarrassment would put me off', 'Test would be uncomfortable', 'Embarrassing', 'Wouldn't want a test in that part of body', 'Discomfort would put me off' and 'Might be painful' (Cronbach's alpha = 0.83).

The remaining measures were as follows. *Fear of cancer* included: 'What will be will be', 'Fear of cancer would put me off', 'Would rather not know' and 'Would make me worry about cancer'. *Screening is not a priority* was made up of 'The test will take up too much time', 'I'm too busy to go for the test' and 'Is no need for healthy people to have the test'. *Knowledge* comprised 'Most people with polyps have no symptoms', 'Removing polyps helps prevent cancer', 'Many people who get cancer are cured', 'The test will reduce the chance of getting bowel cancer' and 'Cancer caught early has a high cure rate.' *Norms* were assessed with questions asking whether partner/children/friends/significant others 'would want you to have the test', 'wouldn't mind whether you had the test or not' or 'would rather you did not have the test'. *Anticipated affective reactions* were measured by asking participants how 'pleased', 'worried', 'relieved' or 'regretful' they would feel if they did not have the test, had the test and no polyps were found, or had the test and a polyp was removed (response options 'Not at all', 'Not very', 'Quite', 'Very'). *State anxiety* was measured by the six-item version of the Spielberger State Trait Anxiety Inventory. *Screening intention* was assessed with the question, 'Realistically, how likely is it that you will attend for Flexi-Scope screening?' ('Very likely', 'Likely', 'Unlikely' or 'Very unlikely').

Results

A total of 1593 participants (53.7 per cent of the sample) returned a completed questionnaire. There were no differences between the intervention and control groups in response rates (53.8 per cent against 53.6 per cent) or in any of the background demographic measures. The booklet had a significant positive impact on intention to attend and all the other measures (Table 6.1). The intervention group had significantly more positive screening attitudes, greater cancer knowledge and a more positive predicted reaction if no polyps were found or a polyp was found and removed, but a significantly more negative prediction for how they would feel if they did not have the test. The control group had significantly greater fear of cancer, were more likely to perceive the FS test as painful or embarrassing, and were more likely to report that screening was not a priority. The booklet also had an impact on perception of social norms, in that the intervention group were significantly more likely to report that significant others would want them to go for the test, and that a higher percentage of people would go for the test if invited. The booklet had no impact on symptoms, anxiety, perceived health, bowel cancer worry, or perceived bowel cancer risk.

4 Discussion: implications for theory, policy and practice

This chapter has described the early stages of a programme of work designed to produce and evaluate a psycho-educational booklet to increase uptake

Table 6.1   Responses in intervention condition (booklet) and control condition (no booklet)

	Booklet (n = 782)	No booklet (n = 811)		
Screening intention			$\chi^2[3] = 35.20$	***
Very likely to attend	42.5%	29.4%		
Likely	50.2%	57.5%		
Unlikely	5.1%	9.5%		
Very unlikely	2.2%	3.6%		
Positive affective reaction score if did not have test	8.74	9.27	$t = 4.11$	***
Positive affective reaction score if had test and no polyps found	14.93	14.67	$t = 2.61$	**
Positive affective reaction score if had test and polyp removed	12.95	12.27	$t = 5.05$	***
Norms score (positive attitudes by others)	8.92	8.53	$t = 2.79$	**
Estimation of percentage of people who would go for test	52.59	46.98	$t = 5.79$	***
Knowledge score	14.92	13.88	$t = 10.01$	***
Positive screening attitude score	28.68	27.81	$t = 5.73$	***
Anticipated embarrassment/ discomfort score	16.53	17.43	$t = 4.64$	***
'Screening is not a priority' score	5.83	6.19	$t = 4.18$	***
Fear of cancer score	8.40	8.75	$t = 2.50$	*

Notes: *p < 0.05   **p < 0.001   ***p < 0.001

of cancer screening. We have found that the intervention had the desired effect on participants' attitudes and beliefs, and significantly increased intention to attend. Later results will show whether this translates into action. As reported earlier in the chapter, health education initiatives are far from consistently effective. Part of the problem, we have argued, is that many health education materials are designed after only minimal preparatory research, use an ad hoc framework rather than established theory, and are evaluated, if at all, by process or outcome, but rarely both.

The present research used the framework of existing, well-established theory for development. It incorporated extensive quantitative and qualitative research to determine the factors associated with screening uptake, and drew on educational theory for content and presentation. The results presented so far concern the first part of the evaluation, that is, the effects of the intervention on attitudes, expectations and intentions. Behavioural outcome data will be available soon. The present results are promising and, if they translate into effective increases in participation, will offer both a useful practical tool and an opportunity to understand the mediating motivational and attitudinal processes. Carefully conducted research needs a strong theoretical framework, and in turn informs the further development of theory. Much of the research on social cognition models draws on cross-sectional studies to try to examine whether attitudes affect behaviour. Our own study will also contribute experimental data, since it will test whether intervening to change screening attitudes and expectations will in turn lead to changes in screening behaviour. It is a large-scale study, the data will be analysed on an intention-to-treat basis, and extensive process data are available, all of which means that it should contribute significantly to testing and developing the theories on which it is based.

As to health policy, we should like to think that our work provides a model for developing and evaluating health education materials. So long as health education resources restrict researchers to conducting little more than quick, inexpensive, preliminary studies before dissemination, it is likely that health education will continue to suffer from low credibility and minimal public and professional support. Good health in the twenty-first century requires investment in human capital to enable and empower individual action for health.

Acknowledgements

The contributions of Kirsten McCaffery, Tamara Taylor, Professor Stephen Sutton, Dr Wendy Atkin and other members of the research team investigating psychosocial aspects of participation in the ICRF/MRC Flexible Sigmoidoscopy Screening Trial are gratefully acknowledged. Funding for the study was provided by the Imperial Cancer Research Fund and the Medical Research Council.

References

American Cancer Society (1996) *Cancer Facts and Figures*. New York: Author.

Arveux, P., Durand, G., Milan, C. *et al.* (1992) Views of a general population on mass screening for colorectal cancer: the Burgundy Study, *Preventive Medicine*, 21: 574–81.

Atkin, W.S., Cusick, J., Northover, J.M.A. and Whynes, D. (1993) Prevention of colorectal cancer by once only sigmoidoscopy, *The Lancet*, 341(8847): 736–40.

Austoker, J. (1994) Cancer prevention in primary care screening for colorectal cancer, *British Medical Journal*, 309: 382–6.

Becker, M.H. (1974) The health belief model and personal health behaviour, *Health Education Monographs*, 2: 324–474.

Blalock, S.J., DeVellis, B.M. and Sandler, R.S. (1987) Participation in fecal occult blood screening: a critical review, *Preventive Medicine*, 16: 9–18.

Brown, M.L., Potosky, A.L., Thompson, G.B. and Kessler, L.G. (1990) The knowledge and use of screening tests for colorectal and prostate cancer: data from the 1987 National Health Interview Survey, *Preventive Medicine*, 19: 562–74.

Byles, J.E., Redman, S.S., Fisher, R.W. and Boyle, C.A. (1995) Effectiveness of two direct-mail strategies to encourage women to have cervical (PAP) smears, *Health Promotion International*, 10(1): 5–16.

Centers for Disease Control (CDC) (1996) From the Centers for Disease Control and Prevention: screening for colorectal cancer – United States, 1992–1993, and new guidelines, *Journal of the American Medical Association*, 275: 830–1.

Charlton, A. (1986) Planning health education materials, *Medical Teacher*, 8(4): 333–42.

Cockburn, J., Thomas, R.J., McLaughlin, S.J. and Reading, D. (1995) Acceptance of screening for colorectal cancer by flexible sigmoidoscopy, *Journal of Medical Screening*, 2: 79–83.

Elwood, M. (1997) New opportunities for colorectal cancer screening, *New Zealand Medical Journal*, 110: 303–4.

Farrands, P.A., Hardcastle, J.D., Chamberlain, J. and Moss, S. (1984) Factors affecting compliance with screening for colorectal cancer, *Community Medicine*, 6: 12–19.

Hardcastle, J.D., Chamberlain, J.O., Robinson, M.H.E. *et al.* (1996) Randomised controlled trial of faecal-occult-blood screening for colorectal cancer, *The Lancet*, 348(9040): 1472–7.

Hardcastle, J.D., Farrands, P.A., Balfour, T.W. *et al.* (1983) Controlled trial of faecal occult blood testing in the detection of colorectal cancer, *The Lancet*, 322(8340): 1–4.

Hart, A.R., Barone, T.L. and Mayberry, J.F. (1997) Increasing compliance with colorectal cancer screening: the development of effective health education, *Health Education Research*, 12: 101–10.

Hart, A.R., Wicks, A.C.B. and Mayberry, J.F. (1995) Colorectal cancer screening in asymptomatic populations, *Gut*, 36: 590–8.

Herbert, C., Launoy, G. and Gignoux, M. (1997) Factors affecting compliance with colorectal cancer screening in France: differences between intention to participate and actual participation, *European Journal of Cancer Prevention*, 6: 44–52.

Hyman, R.B., Baker, S., Ephraim, R., Moadel, A. and Philip, J. (1994) Health belief model variables as predictors of screening mammography utilization, *Journal of Behavioral Medicine*, 17(4): 391–406.

Hynam, K.A., Hart, A.R., Gay, S.P. *et al.* (1995) Screening for colorectal cancer: reasons for refusal of faecal occult blood testing in general practice in England, *Journal of Epidemiology and Community Health*, 49: 84–6.

Klaaborg, K., Madsen, M.S., Sondergaard, O. and Kronberg, O. (1986) Participation in mass screening for colorectal cancer with faecal occult blood test, *Scandinavian Journal of Gastroenterology*, 21: 1180–4.

Kronberg, O., Fenger, C., Olsen, J., Jorgensen, O.D. and Sondergaard, O. (1996) Randomised study of screening for colorectal cancer with faecal-occult-blood test, *The Lancet*, 348: 1467–71.

Macrae, F.A., Hill, D.J., St John, J.B. *et al.* (1984) Predicting colon cancer screening behaviour from health beliefs, *Preventive Medicine*, 13: 115–26.

Macrae, F.A., St John, D.J., Ambikapathy, A., Sharpe, K. and Garner, J.F. (1986) Factors affecting compliance in colorectal cancer screening: results of a study performed in Ballarat, *Medical Journal of Australia*, 144: 621–3.

Mant, D., Fuller, A., Northover, J. *et al.* (1992) Patient compliance with colorectal cancer screening in general practice, *British Journal of General Practice*, 42: 18–20.

Michielutte, R., Bahnson, J., Dignan, M.B. and Schroeder, E.M. (1992) The use of illustrations and narrative text style to improve readability of a health education brochure, *Journal of Cancer Education*, 7(3): 251–60.

Morrow, G.R. and Morrell, C. (1982) Behavioural treatment for anticipatory nausea and vomiting induced by cancer chemotherapy, *New England Journal of Medicine*, 307: 1476–80.

Myers, R.E., Ross, E., Jepson, C. *et al.* (1994) Modeling adherence to colorectal cancer screening, *Preventive Medicine*, 23: 142–51.

Myers, R.E., Ross, E.A., Wolf, T.A. *et al.* (1991) Behavioral interventions to increase adherence in colorectal cancer screening, *Medical Care*, 29: 1039–50.

Neilson, A.R. and Whynes, D.K. (1995) Determinants of persistent compliance with screening for colorectal cancer, *Social Science and Medicine*, 41: 365–74.

Newcomb, P.A., Norfleet, R.G., Storer, B.E., Surawicz, T.S. and Marcus, P.M. (1992) Screening sigmoidoscopy and colorectal cancer mortality, *Journal of the National Cancer Institute*, 84: 1572–5.

Nichols, S., Koch, E., Lallemand, R.C. *et al.* (1986) Randomised trial of compliance with screening for colorectal cancer, *British Medical Journal*, 293: 107–10.

Office for National Statistics (1998) *1996 Mortality Statistics: Cause*, Series DH2, 23. London: The Stationery Office.

Olynyk, J.K., Aquilia, S., Fletcher, D.R. and Dickinson, J.A. (1996) Flexible sigmoidoscopy screening for colorectal cancer in average-risk subjects: a community-based pilot project, *Medical Journal of Australia*, 165: 74–6.

Pye, G., Christie, M., Chamberlain, J., Moss, S.M. and Hardcastle, J.D. (1988) A comparison of methods for increasing compliance within a general practitioner based screening project for colorectal cancer and the effect of practitioner work-load, *Journal of Epidemiology and Community Health*, 42: 66–71.

Selby, J.V., Friedman, G.D., Quesenberry, C.P., Jr and Weiss, N.S. (1992) A case-control study of screening sigmoidoscopy and mortality from colorectal cancer, *New England Journal of Medicine*, 326: 653–7.

Spector, M.H., Applegate, W.B., Olmstead, S.J., DiVasto, P.V. and Skipper, B. (1981) Assessment of attitudes toward Mass Screening for Colorectal Cancer and Polyps, *Preventive Medicine*, 10: 105–9.

Thompson, R.S., Michnich, M.E., Gray, J., Friedlander, L. and Gilson, B. (1986) Maximizing compliance with hemoccult screening for colon cancer in clinical practice, *Medical Care*, 24(10): 904–14.

Vahabi, M. and Ferris, L. (1995) Improving written patient education materials: a review of the evidence, *Health Education Journal*, 54: 99–106.

Vernon, S. (1997) Participation in colorectal cancer screening: a review, *Journal of the National Cancer Institute*, 89: 1406–22.

Wardle, J., Sutton, S., Williamson, S. *et al.* (2000) Psychosocial influences on older adults' interest in participating in bowel cancer screening, *Preventive Medicine*, 31(4): 323–34.

Weller, D.P., Owen, N., Hiller, J.E. and Willson, K. (1995) Colorectal cancer and its prevention: prevalence of beliefs, attitudes, intentions and behaviour, *Australian Journal of Public Health*, 19: 19–23.

SHEINA ORBELL AND
PASCHAL SHEERAN

7

CHANGING HEALTH BEHAVIOURS: THE ROLE OF IMPLEMENTATION INTENTIONS

This chapter will address the role of implementation intentions (Gollwitzer 1993) in promoting health-related behavioural change. Three behaviours will be considered: breast self-examination, vitamin supplement use and cervical screening uptake. All are preventive health behaviours, that is, behaviours performed in the service of preventing either the onset or consequences of disease. Vitamin supplement use and cervical screening uptake may each be regarded as primary prevention measures, serving to prevent disease; breast self-examination is a secondary preventive measure which serves to detect disease early in order to prevent severe consequences. Each is an individual health-related behaviour, which does not require cooperation from others in order to be performed, but requires regular performance in order to be effective. However, while BSE and vitamin supplement use may be regarded as 'private' behaviours, cervical screening uptake involves interaction with the health service.

1 Changing health behaviours: three examples

1.1 Breast self-examination (BSE)

It is estimated that one in nine women will develop breast cancer in their lifetime (American Cancer Society 1993). Breast cancer cannot at present be prevented and its aetiology is poorly understood. However, early detection may increase survival rates following treatment. One method of early detection is to perform a regular breast self-examination, which involves manual palpation by the woman of the breast tissue with the purpose of early detection of breast lumps (Hill *et al.* 1988; GIVO Interdisciplinary Group for Cancer Care Evaluation 1991). Several studies have obtained support for social cognitive variables in predicting BSE (for example Rippetoe and Rogers 1987; Miller *et al.* 1996; Hodgkins and Orbell 1998). However, there is also evidence that in spite of being motivated women may not actually perform it. For instance, Clarke *et al.* (1991) found that although 61 per cent of women who attended a BSE class intended to perform BSE, only 22 per cent had actually done so at follow-up. This suggests that an intervention that focuses on the problem of translating an intention into action, and provides a means of establishing a regular BSE routine, may be valuable.

1.2 Vitamin C supplement use

Adequate vitamin C is important for the prevention of scurvy (National Research Council 1989) and has also been implicated as an antioxidant nutrient associated with a lower risk of heart disease and some cancers (Block *et al.* 1991; Block 1992; Enstrom *et al.* 1992). Low levels of vitamin C intake have been linked to other health indicators, including low socio-economic status (Hargreaves *et al.* 1980; Shapiro *et al.* 1983) and ethnicity (Bowering and Clancy 1986; Koplan *et al.* 1986). Relatively little psychological work has addressed predictors of supplement use. However, in applications of the Theory of Planned Behaviour, Madden *et al.* (1992) found that TPB measures explained 59 per cent of variance in taking supplements over a two-week period, while Warshaw and Davies (1985) found that intentions explained 53 per cent of vitamin intake over one week. These findings suggest that motivational variables are good predictors of behaviour, at least over the shorter term, and imply that this behaviour represents a valuable context for a stringent test of the role of volition in improving consistent supplement use.

1.3 Uptake of the cervical screening test

Cervical cancer is a significant cause of mortality among women and is almost invariably fatal when detected as a cancer in situ (World Health Organization 1986, 1987). It is estimated that, if women were screened every three years, the cervical cancer mortality rate could be reduced by 70–95 per cent (Greenwald and Sondick 1986). Screening for cervical abnormalities (the cervical smear (pap) test) involves microscopic examination of a sample of cells taken from the woman's cervix with the purpose of detecting abnormalities which, if left untreated, may become cancerous. Evidence shows that attendance for cervical screening is less than optimal. A survey conducted by the National Audit Office (1998) indicated that between 10 and 32 per cent of eligible women remain unscreened. Similar figures have been reported in the USA (Hayward *et al.* 1988; Lantz *et al.* 1997; Ruchlin 1997). A number of psychological variables have been studied in relation to cervical screening (see Orbell and Sheeran 1993 for a review) and support has been found for the role of variables from Protection Motivation Theory (Rogers 1975, 1983) and the Health Belief Model (Janz and Becker 1984) in accounting for differences between attenders and non-attenders (Orbell *et al.* 1996; Orbell and Sheeran 1998). The TPB has also been shown to provide moderate prediction of intentions to undergo screening (Hennig and Knowles 1990). However, the only longitudinal study in the area (Orbell and Sheeran 1998) also showed that, among women who intended to undergo cervical screening, just 43 per cent had actually done so one year later, in spite of receiving invitations from their medical practitioner. A psychological intervention study examining promotion of uptake among those who are motivated to attend may therefore be valuable.

2 Theoretical perspective: the Theory of Planned Behaviour and implementation intentions

2.1 The Theory of Planned Behaviour

The starting point for our three interventions was the Theory of Planned Behaviour (Ajzen 1985; Ajzen and Madden 1986) and its predecessor, the Theory of Reasoned Action (Fishbein *et al.* 1980). As we have seen in earlier chapters, these theories outline the social cognitive processes that govern an individual's decision to enact a given behaviour and provide an explanation of how an individual might be motivated to take up a new behaviour. Since many behaviours of interest to health psychology may be novel behaviours for people (for example attending a first cervical cytology test, attending rehabilitation after a heart attack), an understanding of factors that might influence levels of motivation is of considerable applied importance.

Performance or non-performance of a health-related behaviour is presumed by the TPB to be directly predictable from an intention and, under certain circumstances, from perceived behavioural control. The stronger a person's asserted commitment to a behavioural intention (for example 'I strongly agree that I intend to do X'), the more likely it is that the behaviour will be enacted. Ajzen (1991: 181) notes: 'Intentions are assumed to capture the motivational factors that influence a behaviour, they are indicators of how hard people are willing to try, of how much effort they are planning to exert, in order to perform the behaviour'. Reviews of the literature indicate that intentions are satisfactory predictors of behaviour (Ajzen 1991), accounting for between 20 and 30 per cent of the variance in social and health behaviours (Sheppard *et al.* 1988; Randall and Wolff 1994;

Godin and Kok 1996; Sheeran and Orbell 1998). These findings indicate that people who possess a positive intention to act are more likely to act than people who do not possess such an intention, and suggest that interventions that aim to modify intentions by modifying attitude, subjective norm, and perceived behavioural control may be effective in modifying behavioural enactment.

Intentions do not, however, offer perfect prediction of behaviour. A good deal of variance in behaviour remains unexplained since it seems implausible to attribute 70–80 per cent of the variance in behaviour solely to measurement error (cf. Trafimow 1994). In an attempt to clarify the nature of the 'gap' between intention and behaviour, which cannot be readily observed from correlational statistics, Orbell and Sheeran (1998) showed that the greatest source of inconsistency between intention and behaviour was among 'intenders' who failed to turn their 'good intentions' into action. This suggests that by consideration of strategies people might use to turn their intentions into action, it may be possible to improve the predictability of behaviour and, moreover, to modify the relationship between deciding to act and translating that decision into action.

2.2 Implementation intentions

Gollwitzer's (1993) concept of implementation intentions is one such strategy that people might use. Gollwitzer (1990) and Heckhausen (1991) proposed that the decision to perform a given behaviour arises from the deliberation of the pros and cons of action. This motivational phase of goal pursuit parallels that provided by the Theory of Planned Behaviour and culminates in the formation of a goal intention. However, unlike the TPB, Gollwitzer's (1993) approach additionally posited a post-decisional phase of volitional activity during which plans are made to ensure that a decision is acted upon. These plans are labelled implementation intentions and have a *specific form and function* in behavioural enactment. *Implementation intentions* are plans that commit a person to a time and place for enactment of a behavioural intention. Thus, a goal intention ('I intend to do X') may be supplemented by an implementation intention ('I will do X in time and place Y'). Gollwitzer and Brandstätter (1997) provided evidence that the formation of an implementation intention specifying where and when to enact a goal intention increases the likelihood that a goal will be achieved. Students whose goal intention to write a report during the Christmas holiday was supplemented by an implementation intention concerning where and when they would write the report were more than twice as likely to complete their work on time as those who did not form an implementation intention.

In order to appreciate the significance of implementation intentions, it is important to understand *how* they assist in the translation of intentions into action. Many goal intentions in health psychology relate to the problem of initiating performance of an intended behaviour (for example 'I intend to': 'take the pill', 'go for a dental check-up', 'make an appointment for my next cervical smear test', 'go for a swim'). Intentions of this sort may be endlessly postponed because of competing obligations and intentions and, as a result, may never be acted upon, even if one sets a time frame for their completion, such as in the next month (Kuhl and Goschke 1994; cf. Orbell *et al.* 1997). However, by specifying the particular context and the particular time for enacting the intention, that is, by forming an implementation intention ('I intend to go for a swim at the pool on Pond Street on my way home from work tomorrow'), the difficulty in getting started is overcome. Gollwitzer and Brandstätter (1997) provide evidence that goal intentions that are furnished with implementation intentions are more likely to be enacted because by mentally linking a behavioural act with a particular context for its enactment, good opportunities for enactment are less likely to be missed. In one study, subjects who formed implementation intentions regarding the timing, place and method they would use to play a game were able to recall their chosen options with almost perfect accuracy. This suggests that planning behaviour creates strong memory traces that are easily accessible. In a second study, subjects who formed implementation intentions to make counter-arguments at particular points during a video presentation of a person making racist remarks were considerably faster in expressing them than those who were asked only to specify good opportunities. Making an implementation intention, therefore, seems to ensure that when an opportunity for action presents itself, not only will it be rapidly detected but a decisive answer as to whether one should act now or later will be easily retrieved from memory. It is the *linking of behaviour to situation* that accounts for action initiation.

Implementation intentions are thus a powerful mechanism for overcoming the difficulty in getting started in pursuit of a behavioural goal and are presumed to influence the post-decisional phase of goal-directed behaviour, which occurs after the formation of a behavioural intention. There is evidence that some people with positive intentions may spontaneously form implementation intentions, since some of the students in Gollwitzer and Brandstätter's first study had already formed them regarding where and when they would write their reports. In a correlational study in the health domain, Orbell and Sheeran (2000) showed that people undergoing joint replacement surgery who formed implementation intentions about when to initiate everyday activities following surgery, recovered these activities faster than those who did not form implementation intentions. While these studies suggest that some people with positive intentions may, of their own volition, form implementation intentions and therefore translate their intentions into action, the potential utility of implementation intentions lies with those who are motivated to act but do not do so. The experimental studies presented below examined the effects of supplementing an intention with an implementation intention in relation to performance of three important health related behaviours, breast self-examination (Orbell *et al.* 1997), vitamin supplement use (Sheeran and Orbell 1999) and cervical screening uptake (Sheeran and Orbell 2000). Readers are referred to the original articles for full reports of the studies. Several different theoretical aspects of the role of implementation intentions are illustrated in each of the excerpts.

3 The interventions

3.1 Study 1: performance of breast self-examination (BSE) (Orbell et al. 1997)

Method
Participants in Study 1 were 155 women university students and administrative staff (mean age = 21 years). They were invited to take part in an investigation of women's views concerning breast cancer and BSE, and were asked to complete a brief initial questionnaire, and then a second questionnaire one month later. The implementation intention intervention took the form of a questionnaire manipulation, and was compared with a control condition in which the same questions were administered but without the manipulation. Participants were not informed that they were taking part in an experimental study.

Since it was important to demonstrate the effects of implementation intentions among people who were equivalently motivated, motivation was assessed by Theory of Planned Behaviour constructs prior to the manipulation. Seven-point response scales were used. *Intention* was assessed by three items: 'I intend to carry out BSE in the next month', 'I will carry out BSE in the next month' and 'How likely or unlikely is it that you will carry out BSE in the next month?' *Attitude* towards BSE was assessed by four bipolar scales (important–unimportant, beneficial–harmful, undesirable–desirable and foolish–wise). *Subjective norm* was assessed by the item 'Most women my age perform BSE' (likely–unlikely). Five items were used to assess perceived behavioural control: 'Performing BSE in the next month would be easy–difficult', 'Performing BSE in the next month would be under my control–outside of my control', 'I feel capable–incapable of performing BSE in the next month', 'I am confident–unconfident that I could perform BSE in the next month' and 'I am discouraged from performing BSE in the next month because I feel I do not know how to' (agree–disagree). Women were also asked how frequently they had performed BSE *in the last year* (never–often and never–once a week). The follow-up questionnaire was distributed one month later. *BSE performance* during the past month was assessed by the question 'Did you perform BSE in the past month?' A second, open-ended item was included ('How often did you perform BSE during the past month?') so that we could assess the reliability of self-report. In order to examine the effects of implementation intentions on memory for action, a further question asked respondents to report if they had intended to do BSE in the past month but had not, and to write down reasons why they had not. Women who had performed BSE were also asked where and when they had performed it.

Implementation intentions were manipulated as described by Gollwitzer (1993). The following paragraph was added to the intervention group questionnaires and was presented after assessment of TPB variables:

> You are more likely to carry out your intention to perform BSE if you make a decision about when and where you will do so. Many women find it most convenient to perform BSE at the start of the morning or last thing at night, in the bath or shower, or while they are getting dressed in their bedroom or bathroom. Others like to do it in bed before they go to sleep or prior to getting up. Decide now where and when you will perform BSE in the next month and make a commitment to do so.

Results

Longitudinal data were available for an experimental group of 66 and a control group of 89. All scale reliabilities were high, ranging from 0.79 to 0.95, and the two items assessing behaviour were highly correlated ($r = 0.90$). MANOVA established that the two groups did not differ in terms of motivation or past experience prior to the intervention ($F (5, 149) - 0.94$, NS). While the intervention was highly effective overall, with 64 per cent of women in the intervention group performing BSE compared with just 14 per cent in the control group (chi-square = 37.68, $p < 0.01$), the effects are most strikingly apparent if one examines the effects of implementation intentions among those who had positive intentions to perform BSE prior to the intervention. All the women (100 per cent) who had positive intentions and formed an implementation intention performed BSE, compared with 53 per cent of women who had positive intentions but were not asked to form implementation intentions.

The study also investigated the effects of implementation intentions on memory for intentions, since this is how implementation intentions are proposed to exert their effects. One month after forming their implementation intentions, participants were asked to report where and when they had performed BSE (for example last thing at night in the shower). All but one respondent reported carrying out the behaviour exactly when and where they had initially specified. These findings lend powerful support to the argument that implementation intentions are readily accessible in memory. Furthermore, the correspondence of time and place supports the proposition that implementation intentions direct behaviour in a relatively automatic manner. Finally, examination of the reasons given for non-performance of BSE by those who intended but did not act revealed that the most frequently reported reason was 'I forgot', which was endorsed by 70 per cent of abstainers in the control group. Overall, these findings are consistent with the theoretical proposition that implementation intentions direct behaviour by ensuring that opportunities for action are not missed.

3.2 Study 2: vitamin supplement use (Sheeran and Orbell 1999, Study 1)

Method
Participants in Study 2 were 103 undergraduates selected at random from two university halls of residence. Their mean age was 18.8 years and 56 per cent of the sample were women. Participants were asked to take part in a study concerned with taking vitamin C tablets and were given a sealed bottle containing 50 tablets. They were informed that they would be asked to complete two further questionnaires. Half the sample were assigned at random to the intervention condition, half to a non-intervention control condition, but participants were not told of the experimental nature of the study. The researcher was blind to each participant's allocation.

The design in this study was similar to that in the BSE intervention. However, we also wanted to provide empirical evidence that the effects of implementation intentions on behaviour were not attributable to changes in motivation occurring after forming an implementation intention. Study 2 therefore included three phases of data collection. At Time 1, motivation was assessed using Theory of Planned Behaviour measures. The implementation intention manipulation was included at the end of the Time 1 questionnaire, as in Study 1. Ten days later intention was reassessed in order to establish that the manipulation had not increased intention to use supplements. Final behaviour was assessed at Time 3.

Seven-point response scales were employed for all measures, unless specified otherwise. *Intention* to use supplements was measured by two items: 'I intend to take a vitamin C tablet every day for the next three weeks' and 'I will take a vitamin C tablet every day for the next three weeks.' *Attitude* was assessed by seven bipolar scales ('good–bad', 'pleasant–unpleasant', 'healthy–unhealthy', 'nice–nasty', 'sensible–foolish', 'harmful–beneficial', 'useful–useless') and the item 'I think that taking one vitamin C tablet per day would increase my resistance to common infections' ('agree–disagree'). *Subjective norm* was measured by the item 'Most people whose opinion matters to me think I should take a vitamin C tablet every day' (agree–disagree). Four items were used to assess *perceived behavioural control*: 'For me, taking a vitamin C tablet every day for the next three weeks would be . . . (easy–difficult), 'How many obstacles are there that would prevent you taking a vitamin C tablet every day for the next three weeks?' (numerous obstacles would prevent me–few obstacles would prevent me), 'How much control do you think you have over whether or not you take a vitamin C tablet every day for the next three weeks?' (complete control–no control) and 'How confident are you that you will be able to take a vitamin C tablet every day for the next three weeks?' (confident–unconfident). *Past behaviour* was measured by the item 'How often in the past have you taken vitamin C tablets?' (five-point scale, 'never–always'). *Follow-up behaviour* was assessed at both Time 2 and Time 3 by self-report ('How many vitamin C tablets have you taken in the past 11 days?') and by a pill count performed by the researcher. In order to control for absences, participants were also asked to indicate how many days they had been away.

Implementation intentions were assessed in a manner similar to that for Study 1. Participants in the intervention condition were asked to specify where and when they would take a vitamin C tablet every day for the next three weeks. The intervention was delivered at the end of the Time 1 questionnaire, following completion of TPB measures:

> You are more likely to carry out your intention to take a vitamin C tablet every day for the next 3 weeks if you make a decision about where and when you will do so. Decide now where and when you will take the vitamin C tablets in the next 3 weeks. You may find it useful to take a tablet just before or just after something else that you do regularly, such as brushing your teeth. Please write in below where and when you will take a vitamin C tablet every day for the next 3 weeks (e.g. in my room at 7pm just after my evening meal).

Results
Reliability for each of the measures was satisfactory, ranging from 0.71 to 0.78. MANOVA showed that participants in the experimental and control conditions did not differ in terms of attitude, subjective norm, perceived behavioural control or past behaviour ($F_{(5, 72)} = 0.20$, NS). Nor were there any differences in gender or age between the two groups. Moreover, intentions were strong in both groups with mean scores above 6.0 on the 1–7 point scale. From these findings it can be concluded that the intervention and control groups were initially equally motivated to take a vitamin C tablet every day for three weeks.

Table 7.1 shows the results of the intervention, measured by number of pills missed over a three-week period. At Time 2, ten days after the intervention, both the pill count and self-report showed no significant differences between the two groups on the numbers of missed tablets. By Time 3, however, the intervention group had missed significantly fewer pills than the control group, according to both self-report ($t = 2.05$, $p < 0.05$) and pill

Table 7.1   Number of pills missed by implementation intention and control groups (Study 2)

	Implementation intention group	Control group
Time 3		
Pill count	1.57	3.53
Self-report	2.68	4.85
Time 2		
Pill count	0.61	1.00
Self-report	0.92	1.43

Note: adapted from Sheeran and Orbell 1999

count (t = 1.86, p < 0.05). The self-report and pill count measures correlated strongly (r = 0.90 and 0.92 for the experimental and control groups respectively).

The findings indicate that the implementation intention intervention was successful in ensuring that vitamin C tablets were taken by participants. In order to ensure that the manipulation had not achieved its effects by altering motivation to take the pills, we compared changes in the intention measure across time for the intervention and control groups. Consistent with the proposal that the findings could not be explained by motivational factors, the experimental and control groups did not differ in their intentions (F (1, 76) = 2.93, NS), nor were there significant changes across time (F (1, 76) = 1.39, NS) or a significant interaction between condition and time (F (1, 76) = 0.38, NS).

3.3 Study 3: attendance at a cervical screening test (Sheeran and Orbell 2000)

Method

Study 3 concerns the role of implementation intentions in increasing the likelihood of attending for a cervical screening test after having been sent an invitation. Participants were a general population sample of 114 women registered at a general practice in England (mean age = 40.62 years). All were eligible for a cervical screening test and were sent a standard postcard reminder by their medical practitioner. They were then sent a confidential questionnaire concerning their views of the cervical smear test. The implementation intention intervention was contained unobtrusively in the questionnaires sent to the intervention group participants.

Whereas Studies 1 and 2 reported above considered relatively simple goal intentions where it was necessary only to specify where and when to perform the behaviour specified in the goal intention ('I intend to do X in time and place Y'), attendance for a cervical smear test requires a more complex form of implementation intention. Since, in order to attend for a cervical smear test, it is first necessary to make an appointment, it was theorized that an implementation intention would need to specify an act in the service of a goal intention ('I intend to do Z in time and place Y in order to achieve behavioural goal X'). Thus, in this third study, we examined the effects of a more complex implementation intention on the likelihood of achieving a behavioural goal.

Theory of Planned Behaviour measures were each assessed on five-point scales. *Intention* was measured by two items: 'I intend to go for a cervical smear within the next three months' and 'I will try to go for a cervical smear within the next three months' (strongly agree–strongly disagree). *Attitude* was assessed by eight scales (not at all–extremely) in response to the stem 'For me, going for a cervical smear within the next three months would be . . . worthwhile, worrying, reassuring, embarrassing, wise, healthy, unpleasant, important'. *Subjective norm* was assessed by the item 'Most people who are important to me think that I should go for a cervical smear in the next three months' (strongly agree–strongly disagree). *Perceived behavioural control* was measured by three items: 'How easy or difficult would it be for you to go for a cervical smear within the next three months?' (very easy–very difficult), 'How confident are you that you will be able to go for a cervical smear within the next three months?' (very confident–very unconfident) and 'If I wanted to, I could easily go for a cervical smear within the next three months' (strongly agree–strongly disagree). *Behaviour* was reliably determined from participants' medical records.

As in Studies 1 and 2, there were two conditions: intervention and control. Participants in the intervention condition were asked to form an implementation intention specifying when, where and how they would make an appointment to go for a cervical smear test in the next three months:

> You are more likely to go for a cervical smear if you decide when and where you will go. Please write down in the space below when, where and how you will make an appointment.

Results

MANOVA confirmed that there were no differences between the intervention and control groups for TPB measures, age or previous screening behaviours ($F (8, 105) = 1.51$, NS). Intentions were positive in both conditions, with mean scores above 4 on a 1–5 scale, indicating that both groups were highly motivated to attend for screening prior to the experimental manipulation.

The effect of the implementation intention manipulation on behaviour was analysed by cross tabulating condition with attendance. The effect was highly significant (chi-square = 9.20, $p < 0.01$): 69 per cent of the control group attended for screening, a higher figure than obtained in many previous studies (see for example Orbell and Sheeran 1998); but, most impressively, the figure for the intervention group was 92 per cent. These findings provide convincing evidence that implementation intention formation makes participants more likely to succeed in keeping an important health-check appointment.

4 Discussion: implications for theory, policy and practice

Theories such as the Theory of Planned Behaviour provide an adequate account of motivation to perform health-related behaviour, and offer a valuable basis for interventions to modify people's motivation to act, by modifying attitude, subjective norm and perceived behavioural control. However, the relationship between deciding to undertake a health action and then doing so is less than perfect, and many people who are positively motivated do not translate their 'good intentions' into action (Orbell and Sheeran 1998). Implementation intentions (Gollwitzer 1993) provide a simple and parsimonious solution to the problem of getting started in performing a novel health action. The three experiments reported above show that the simple formation of an implementation intention specifying where and when to perform a focal behaviour dramatically increased the likelihood of performance among people who were positively motivated. The fact that this effect was obtained across three different behaviours, using both self-report and objective behavioural indices, and among both student and general population samples, confirms the generalisability of the findings to related health behaviours.

The findings also have a number of theoretical implications. The effects of implementation intentions demonstrated in these studies were obtained among samples shown to be initially equally motivated to act. Moreover, measures of intention taken after the intervention demonstrated that forming an implementation intention did not alter motivation. These findings support the proposition that implementation intentions, rather than being a tool of persuasion, are a tool of implementation, which influences post decisional cognitive processes. Studies by Orbell *et al.* (1997) and Sheeran and Orbell (1999) have demonstrated that implementation intentions work by affecting memory processes, while Orbell and Sheeran (2000) have shown that the formation of implementation intentions leads to faster action initiation. Linking a specific act to a specific context for its performance ensures that, when the situation is encountered, the behaviour comes swiftly to mind and is unlikely to be forgotten.

Initiating a new health-related behaviour often requires overcoming competing intentions and obligations. Implementation intentions are useful not only for initiating a single act (Orbell *et al.* 1997; Orbell and Sheeran 2000;

Sheeran and Orbell 2000), but also for establishing regular or routine performance of a new behaviour that needs to be repeated regularly in order to be effective (Sheeran and Orbell 1999). Our findings also suggest that, in order to achieve the focal behaviour, it is sometimes necessary first to form an implementation intention to enact a behaviour *in the service of* the focal behaviour (Sheeran and Orbell 2000). Thus, while our studies demonstrate the value of implementation intentions in improving the likelihood of performing BSE, taking vitamin C supplements and attending for a cervical smear test, and make an important contribution to understanding these health-related behaviours, the findings also argue for the value of augmenting social cognitive accounts of health-related behaviour generally, to include greater attention to the role of volition.

References

Ajzen, I. (1985) From intentions to actions: a theory of planned behaviour, in J. Kuhl and J. Beckman (eds) *Action Control: From Cognition to Behaviour*. Heidelberg: Springer.

Ajzen, I. (1991) The Theory of Planned Behavior, *Organizational Behavior and Human Decision Processes*, 50: 179–211.

Ajzen, I. and Madden, T.J. (1986) Prediction of goal-directed behavior: attitudes, intention, and perceived behavioral control, *Journal of Experimental Social Psychology*, 22: 453–74.

American Cancer Society (1993) *Cancer Facts and Figures*. New York: Author.

Block, G. (1992) Vitamin C and reduced mortality, *Epidemiology*, 3: 189–91.

Block, G., Hensen, D.E. and Levine, M. (1991) Vitamin C: a new look, *Annals of Internal Medicine*, 114: 909–10.

Bowering, J. and Clancy, K.L. (1986) Nutritional status of children in relation to vitamin and mineral use, *Journal of the American Dietetic Association*, 86: 1033–8.

Clarke, V., Hill, D., Rassaby, J., White, V. and Hirst, S. (1991) Determinants of continued breast self-examination practice in women 40 years and over after personalised instruction, *Health Education Research*, 6: 297–306.

Enstrom, J.E., Kanim, L.E. and Klein, M.A. (1992) Vitamin C intake and mortality among a sample of the United States population, *Epidemiology*, 3: 194–202.

Fishbein, M., Ajzen, I. and McArdle, J. (1980) Changing the behavior of alcoholics: effects of persuasive communication, in I. Ajzen and M. Fishbein (eds) *Understanding Attitudes and Predicting Social Behavior*. Englewood Cliffs, NJ: Prentice-Hall.

GIVO Interdisciplinary Group for Cancer Care Evaluation (1991) Practice of breast self-examination: disease extent at diagnosis and patterns of surgical care: a report from an Italian study, *Journal of Epidemiology and Community Health*, 45: 112–16.

Godin, G. and Kok, G. (1996) The Theory of Planned Behavior: a review of its applications to health-related behaviors, *American Journal of Health Promotion*, 11(2): 87–98.

Gollwitzer, P.M. (1990) Action phases and mind-sets, in E.T. Higgins and R.M. Sorrentino (eds) *Handbook of Motivation and Cognition: Foundations of Social Behavior*, 2. New York: Guilford.

Gollwitzer, P.M. (1993) Goal achievement: the role of intentions, in W. Stroebe and M. Hewstone (eds) *European Review of Social Psychology*, 4. Chichester: Wiley.

Gollwitzer, P.M. and Brandstätter, V. (1997) Implementation intentions and effective goal pursuit, *Journal of Personality and Social Psychology*, 73(1): 186–99.

Greenwald, P. and Sondick, E.J. (1986) *Cancer Control Objectives for the Nation: 1985–2000*. Bethesda, MD: National Cancer Institute.

Hargreaves, M.K., Baquet, C. and Gamshadzahi, A. (1980) Diet, nutritional status, and cancer risk in American Blacks, *Nutrition and Cancer*, 12: 1–28.

Hayward, R.A., Shapiro, M.F., Freeman, H.E. and Corey, R. (1988) Who gets screened for cervical and breast cancer? Results from a national survey, *Archives of Internal Medicine*, 148: 1177–81.

Heckhausen, H. (1991) *Motivation and Action*. Berlin: Springer-Verlag.

Hennig, P. and Knowles, A. (1990) Factors influencing women over 40 years to take precautions against cervical cancer, *Journal of Applied Social Psychology*, 20: 1612–21.

Hill, D., White, V., Jolley, D. and Mapperson, K. (1988) Self-examination of the breast: is it beneficial? Meta-analysis of studies investigating breast self-examination and extent of disease in patients with breast cancer, *British Medical Journal*, 297: 271–5.

Hodgkins, S. and Orbell, S. (1998) Does protection-motivation theory predict behaviour? A longitudinal study exploring the role of past behaviour, *Psychology and Health*, 13: 237–50.

Janz, N. and Becker, M.H. (1984) The health belief model: a decade later, *Health Education Quarterly*, 11: 1–47.

Koplan, J.P., Annest, J.L., Layde, P.M. and Rubin, G.L. (1986) Nutrient intake and supplementation in the United States (NHANES II), *American Journal of Public Health*, 76: 287–9.

Kuhl, J. and Goschke, T. (1994) State orientation and the activation and retrieval of intentions in memory, in J. Kuhl and J. Beckmann (eds) *Volition and Personality*. Seattle, WA: Hogrefe and Huber.

Lantz, P.M., Weigers, M.E. and House, J.S. (1997) Education and income differentials in breast and cervical cancer screening, *Medical Care*, 35: 219–326.

Madden, T.J., Ellen, P.S. and Ajzen, I. (1992) A comparison of the theory of planned behavior and the theory of reasoned action, *Personality and Social Psychology Bulletin*, 18: 3–9.

Miller, S.M., Shoda, Y. and Hurley, K. (1996) Applying cognitive-social theory to health-protective behaviour: breast self-examination in cancer screening, *Psychological Bulletin*, 119: 70–94.

National Audit Office (1998) *The Performance of the National Health Service Cervical Screening Programme in England*. London: National Audit Office.

National Research Council (1989) *Recommended Dietary Allowances*, 10th edn. Washington, DC: National Academy Press.

Orbell, S. and Sheeran, P. (1993) Health psychology and uptake of preventive health services: a review of 30 years' research on cervical screening, *Psychology and Health*, 8: 417–33.

Orbell, S. and Sheeran, P. (1998) 'Inclined abstainers': a problem for predicting health-related behaviour, *British Journal of Social Psychology*, 37: 151–65.

Orbell, S. and Sheeran, P. (2000) Motivational and volitional processes in action initiation: a field study of implementation intentions, *Journal of Applied Social Psychology*, 30: 780–97.

Orbell, S., Crombie, I. and Johnston, G. (1996) Social cognition and social structure in the prediction of cervical screening uptake, *British Journal of Health Psychology*, 1: 35–50.

Orbell, S., Hodgkins, S. and Sheeran, P. (1997) Implementation intentions and the theory of planned behavior, *Personality and Social Psychology Bulletin*, 23(9): 945–54.

Randall, D.M. and Wolff, J.A. (1994) The time interval in the intention-behaviour relationship: meta-analysis, *British Journal of Social Psychology*, 33: 405–18.

Rippetoe, P.A. and Rogers, R.W. (1987) Effects of components of protection-motivation theory on adaptive and maladaptive coping with a health threat, *Journal of Personality and Social Psychology*, 52(3): 596–604.

Rogers, R.W. (1975) A protection motivation theory of fear appeals and attitude change, *Journal of Psychology*, 91: 93–114.

Rogers, R.W. (1983) Cognitive and physiological processes in fear appeals and attitude change, in J.T. Cacioppo and R.E. Petty (eds) *Social Psychophysiology*. New York: Guilford.

Ruchlin, H.S. (1997) Prevalence and correlates of breast and cervical screening among older women, *Obstetrics and Gynaecology*, 90: 16–21.

Shapiro, L.R., Samuels, S., Breslow, L. and Camacho, T. (1983) Patterns of vitamin C intake from food and supplements: survey of an adult population in Alameda county, California, *American Journal of Public Health*, 73: 773–8.

Sheeran, P. and Orbell, S. (1998) Do intentions predict condom use? Meta-analysis and examination of six moderator variables, *British Journal of Social Psychology*, 37: 231–50.

Sheeran, P. and Orbell, S. (1999) Implementation intentions and repeated behaviour: augmenting the predictive validity of the theory of planned behaviour, *European Journal of Social Psychology*, 29: 349–69.

Sheeran, P. and Orbell, S. (2000) Using implementation intentions to increase attendance for cervical cancer screening, *Health Psychology*, 19(3): 283–9.

Sheppard, B.H., Hartwick, J. and Warshaw, P.R. (1988) The Theory of Reasoned Action: a meta-analysis of past research with recommendations for modifications and future research, *Journal of Consumer Research*, 15: 325–39.

Trafimow, D. (1994) Predicting intentions to use a condom from perceptions of normative pressure and confidence in those perceptions, *Journal of Applied Social Psychology*, 24: 2151–63.

Warshaw, P.R. and Davis, F.D. (1985) Disentangling behavioural intention and behavioural expectation, *Journal of Experimental Social Psychology*, 21(3): 213–28.

World Health Organization (1986) Control of cancer of the cervix uteri, *Bulletin of the World Health Organization*, 64: 607–18.

World Health Organization (1987) Genital human papillomavirus infections and cancer: memorandum from a WHO meeting, *Bulletin of the World Health Organization*, 65: 817–27.

8

DIANNE PARKER

CHANGING DRIVERS' ATTITUDES TO SPEEDING: USING THE THEORY OF PLANNED BEHAVIOUR

Driving with excess speed is a serious social problem, as speeding is known to contribute causally to, or at least worsen the effects of, many road traffic accidents. Considerable efforts have been made in recent years to employ physical and/or technological means to slow drivers down. However, such measures are unlikely to result in permanent behaviour change while speeding is still regarded as acceptable behaviour by many drivers. One way to change these perceptions would be to develop publicity and road safety campaigns grounded in the theoretical principles of the psychology of attitude change. This chapter describes one attempt to use those principles. An extended version of Ajzen's (1985) Theory of Planned Behaviour was used in a study of the beliefs, values and attitudes that underpin the decision to speed in a 30 m.p.h. zone. Those beliefs were then targeted in a video-based attitude change intervention. The results show that theory-based interventions have the potential to bring about statistically significant attitude change, and so might profitably be used to guide the development of future road safety campaigns.

1 Changing drivers' attitudes to speeding

It is a commonplace that road traffic accidents are a serious social problem. In 1998 there were a total of 238,923 recorded road traffic accidents in Great Britain, resulting in 325,212 casualties. Of those casualties, over 44,000 were seriously injured, and 3421 were killed (Department of the Environment, Transport and the Regions (DETR) 1999). Certain groups are particularly vulnerable. For example, among young men between the ages of 20 and 29, road traffic accidents are the most common cause of death, accounting for 19 per cent of all fatalities in that age group. In recent years parents' concerns about the hazards of traffic have contributed to the restriction of children's freedom to play, and many elderly people are fearful of negotiating traffic as either a pedestrian or a driver.

Driving with excess speed is a major contributory factor in many road traffic accidents. There is reliable evidence from a number of countries that excess speed increases the risk of accident involvement. An early study by Sabey and Staughton (1975) in which British accident reports were analysed concluded that driving too fast was second only to drink-driving as the most important cause of accidents. Similarly, a cross-sectional analysis of official US data in 1987 showed speed to be directly related to motor-vehicle death rates (Zlatoper 1991); a more recent study in British Columbia (Cooper 1997) showed that convictions for both 'excessive speed' and 'exceeding the speed limit' were predictive of subsequent culpable crash involvement. Nor are speed-related accidents confined to high speed roads. The statistics for Britain in 1998 show that 65 per cent of all accidents, and around 34 per cent of all fatal road traffic accidents, occurred on roads with a 30 m.p.h. speed limit (DETR 1999). Even allowing for the fact that most driving is done on such minor roads, a disproportionate number of accidents occur on them. Thus the accident rate per 100 million vehicle kilometres in 1998 was 71 for minor roads, compared to 52 for A roads and 11 for motorways (DETR 1999).

In spite of these statistics, exceeding the speed limit on 30 m.p.h. roads is not regarded as a serious, or even socially unacceptable, road traffic offence by many. A survey for the Scottish Office (System Three 1997) showed that drivers feel that the likelihood of detection, injury or damage, or social opprobrium following 'moderate speeding' is low. In a self-report survey, 88 per cent of drivers readily admitted to speeding at 40 m.p.h. on 30 m.p.h. zones 'at least sometimes' (Corbett and Simon 1992).

Several types of intervention strategies have been employed in attempts to reduce the frequency and extent of speeding on the roads. One approach involves changing the physical driving environment, although the available data suggest that reductions in speed following the introduction of radar detectors or speed cameras are temporary and confined to the specific area in which the equipment operates (Casey and Lund 1993; Teed *et al.* 1993; Corbett 1995). Moreover, while traffic-calming measures such as speed humps and road narrowing can be successful in reducing average speeds, it is not practical to apply such engineering solutions on all roads (Schnuell and Lange 1992; Zaidel *et al.* 1992).

An alternative strategy involves increased enforcement of speed limits by the police, but this is expensive and the evidence suggests that the beneficial effects are short-lived once enforcement returns to pre-intervention levels (Holland and Conner 1996; Vaa 1997). It has also been suggested, in a field experiment among Dutch drivers, that enforcement of the motorway speed limit serves to deter those who are already non-speeders rather than to change the behaviour of those who do break the limit (de Waard and Rooijers 1994).

A report by the Parliamentary Advisory Council for Traffic Safety (PACTS) reviewed the research evidence on the factors that influence drivers to speed and concluded that enforcement plays a less important role than social pressure, and that consequently 'mechanisms to encourage and support social pressures to conform to the law are needed' (PACTS 1999). Many anti-speeding interventions attempt to provide such a mechanism by trying to persuade drivers not to exceed the speed limit. Expensive anti-speeding publicity campaigns disseminated through the media are commonplace in most countries. However, it is often the case that the content of such campaigns owes more to the imagination and inspiration of the advertising agency than to the theoretical principles of the psychology of attitude change.

Since 1988, in a research programme carried out at the University of Manchester and funded by the DETR, we have tried to apply those principles to the problem of speeding drivers. We have investigated the usefulness of the Theory of Planned Behaviour for the development and targeting of anti-speeding messages. The aim has been to apply the TPB framework to a range of driving violations, including speeding, with a view to identifying the beliefs and values that distinguish those drivers who report committing violations (Parker *et al.* 1992, 1995).

2 Theoretical perspective: the Theory of Planned Behaviour

As this volume attests, the Theory of Reasoned Action (Fishbein and Ajzen 1975) and subsequently the TPB (Ajzen and Fishbein 1980; Ajzen 1985) have been very popular with applied social psychologists studying a wide range of health-promoting behaviours, including smoking (Budd 1986; Grube *et al.* 1986), contraceptive use (Boyd and Wandersman 1991), seat-belt use (Budd *et al.* 1984), drinking (Schlegel *et al.* 1977; Kilty 1978), dental behaviour (McCaul *et al.* 1988; Beale and Manstead 1991), infant feeding (Manstead *et al.* 1983), health screening (Ronis and Kaiser 1989; Brubaker and Fowler 1990) and AIDS-preventive behaviour (Terry *et al.* 1993).

One reason for the popularity of the model is that it offers a relatively simple theoretical account of the links between attitudes, intentions and behaviour, together with clear specification of how those contructs should be operationalized. In addition, it is theoretically possible to identify the specific beliefs that are important predictors of intentions and behaviour, and to use them to guide the content of behaviour change interventions. However, although the model has been widely used to specify the attitudinal determinants of many health behaviours, as noted by Conner and Sparks (1996), rather fewer attempts have been made to assess the efficacy of interventions based on the model. The need for such studies was articulated by Martin Fishbein in his foreword to an edited volume reporting the application of the model to AIDS-preventive behaviour.

> The ultimate test of the utility of the theory of reasoned action will rest upon its ability to guide the development of effective behavior change interventions . . . the present volume only holds out the promise of effective interventions. Perhaps the next step for the Editors of this book is to compile a volume describing tests of the theory 'in action', by presenting a number of studies evaluating the effectiveness of theory-based interventions.
>
> (Fishbein, in Terry *et al.* 1993: xiv)

In the programme of research reported here efforts were made to develop and evaluate a theory-based intervention of the kind Fishbein suggested. In an initial study utilizing the TPB (Parker *et al.* 1992) hierarchical multiple regression analyses showed that attitude to behaviour, subjective norm and perceived behavioural control all performed reasonably well in predicting intention to commit a range of driving violations, including speeding at 40 m.p.h. in a 30 m.p.h. zone. Subsequently, multivariate analyses of variance were employed to uncover those specific beliefs that differentiated 'intenders' from 'non-intenders'.

It was found that in terms of the attitudinal component, which concerns the driver's beliefs about the likely consequences of their committing the violation in question, it was beliefs concerning the likelihood of being stopped by the police, causing an accident, and putting pedestrians at risk that distinguished those more and less likely to speed. In terms of the normative component, which reflects how mindful the driver is of the approval (or disapproval) of others, the perceived expectations of partners, close family and same-sex friends distinguished those more and less likely to commit a violation. Perceived behavioural control was also important, such that the less control drivers reported feeling over their own driving behaviour, the lower were their reported intentions to refrain from committing violations. These, then, were the beliefs to be included in a subsequent intervention.

In a second study (Parker *et al.* 1995), in which the TPB was applied to a further set of driving violations, two additional predictor variables were included. These were measures of moral norm and anticipated regret, which were included to reflect aspects of the individual's personal normative beliefs about the behaviour. Specifically, moral norm reflects the individual's personal internalized moral rules and has been shown to be a valuable addition to the TPB in studies of behaviours with moral implications (for example Schwartz and Tessler 1972; Pomazal and Jaccard 1976; Zuckerman and Reis 1978; Gorsuch and Ortberg 1983). Anticipated regret, which reflects the negative affect an individual might anticipate following risky behaviour, has been shown to be important in predicting behavioural expectations about sexual and contraceptive behaviour (Richard *et al.* 1996). These two additional predictors were included because the commission of driving violations is inherently risky, and may also have a moral dimension, for some drivers at least. The addition of these two new personal norm variables significantly improved the predictive performance of the model. Furthermore, they both distinguished drivers who were relatively more likely to violate than others, such that high violators endorsed more strongly the belief that 'It would be quite wrong to [commit a violation]', and endorsed less strongly the belief that committing a violation would 'make me feel good'. For that reason it was decided to include personal norm in the intervention study.

3 The intervention

3.1 Method

On the basis of the survey results, a series of short videos were made, each of which was designed to change beliefs, attitudes and intentions in relation to speeding at 40 m.p.h. in a residential area governed by a 30 m.p.h. speed limit. The main aim of the study was to assess the effectiveness of videos based on clusters of beliefs identified as important by the TPB studies. Each video was focused on one such cluster of beliefs.

The videos were made, under our direction, by a professional audiovisual design company based in Manchester. Working with an extremely limited budget, they produced four short videos for us, each targeting one of the four key concepts outlined above. All four videos were of similar length, featured the same actors and the same car, and were shot in the same location. The road used was chosen because it was a good example of the type of residential street, with cars parked on both sides, that had been referred to as the context for the speeding violation in our earlier empirical study. The main character, Tom, was played by an actor in his late twenties.

The normative beliefs video was designed to convey to the viewer the message that people do not like being driven by a speeding driver. Our previous research showed that drivers who report intending to speed are less likely than non-intenders to believe that their partners, their same-sex friends and/or their immediate family disapprove of their driving in this way. Each of those people/groups therefore appeared in the video, and was seen to express disapproval of Tom's speeding behaviour.

The behavioural beliefs video was intended to show that a quiet residential road can, in fact, be an obstacle course of hazards. Our earlier research had shown that those who intend to speed believe less strongly than others that speeding would result in being stopped and fined, would cause an accident, or would put the lives of pedestrians at risk. This video therefore showed Tom driving down the road and encountering each of those potential hazards. The objective of the video was to make the audience think about what could have happened, introducing the idea that such hazards *are* likely to be present on seemingly innocuous residential roads, and showing that by keeping to the speed limit you can increase your chances of being able to deal with whatever hazards do arise.

In the perceived behavioural control video Tom was confronted with what we regard as the two main components of behavioural control. The first sequence was designed to illustrate the notion of control over *internal* promptings, in the sense of resisting temptation. In the second sequence the notion of control over external pressure was introduced. When Tom complains about feeling pressured by the car behind, a warning voice reminds him that it is his *own* foot on the accelerator, and that he is free to choose his own driving speed. This video was designed to persuade the audience that the driver can control their own behaviour, and that it is not impossible to keep to the speed limit.

The video featuring anticipated regret was the most difficult to develop, as it attempted to portray speeding as inherently wrong, as the sort of thing that would lead to a driver feeling guilty or ashamed if they were to do it. Given that many drivers do not see speeding as socially unacceptable behaviour, this was a difficult idea to convey. The aim was to persuade viewers that if they do speed on a residential road, they should feel bad about it, because speeding is inherently wrong and unacceptable behaviour, whether or not there are serious negative consequences. The video showed an elderly woman, startled by a speeding car, being helped across the road by Tom, who sympathizes and commiserates with her. Later Tom, glancing at his own speedometer, and realizing that now he is speeding, slows down to avoid being the type of driver he was earlier seen condemning.

3.2 Qualitative results

The impact of the videos was assessed both qualitatively and quantitatively. Focus groups of between 4 and 8 drivers were used to promote discussion of the videos in terms of both content and impact. Other participants took part in the quantitative assessment, which was carried out by means of a questionnaire administered to a quota sample of 238 drivers. Table 8.1 shows the age and gender breakdown of the participants in the quantitative assessment.

Small groups of drivers viewed one of the four videos twice, after which they were given three minutes in which to list the thoughts that had occurred to them while watching it. This standard thought-listing measure was taken because attitude change theory argues that it is important to assess the

Table 8.1 Quantitative assessment: numbers of drivers by age-group, sex, and type of video seen

Video	Sex	17–24 years	25–32 years	33–40 years	Total
Normative beliefs	Male	7	7	7	21
	Female	9	7	8	24
Behavioural beliefs	Male	7	8	7	22
	Female	8	8	7	23
Perceived behavioural control	Male	7	9	7	23
	Female	8	8	9	25
Anticipated regret	Male	8	8	7	23
	Female	8	10	9	27
Control	Male	11	7	7	25
	Female	9	7	9	25
Total		82	79	77	238

participants' cognitive responses to a persuasive message. This is because bringing about lasting attitude change depends on making people think through the implications of the message in order to assimilate it. The thoughts listed were classified by two independent judges into one of five categories: anti-speeding, pro-speeding, anti-video, pro-video and neutral. For each video, the number of anti-speeding thoughts outweighed the number of pro-speeding thoughts, giving reason to believe that all four videos would have the potential to evoke attitude change.

Further qualitative assessment through focus groups showed that some participants had clearly got the main message of the videos they watched. The following quotations are examples.

Behavioural beliefs:

> I suppose it was that even on a road like this, there are hazards . . . on an 'all's quiet' sort of road where you don't expect kids to run out or people to open a door, but it does happen.

Normative beliefs:

> There's this guy and you hear everything his friends say about him, and it sort of says to you, do you know what your friends think of you?

Perceived behavioural control:

> I think it makes people aware . . . that they have a responsibility . . . a kind of like a personal challenge.

Anticipated regret:

It shows that most people who drive say 'I wouldn't do that' then he actually looks at his clock and realizes how fast he was going, but until that point he didn't think about it.

However, some of the themes that seemed to run through the group discussions illustrated the difficulties of achieving real attitude change. Drivers seemed to want to shift responsibility for their behaviour behind the wheel onto the shoulders of others: the police, pedestrians, or even the car itself. The following quotations are relevant to the concept of perceived behavioural control.

Most of the roads I travel down, there's a 30 m.p.h. limit. The traffic rate is a steady 40 m.p.h., and that's the steady flow both ways, and the police are just obvious by their absence. They must be condoning it, you know, want to increase the traffic flow.

Well, you think that the woman was in the wrong spot for trying to cross over at that particular spot.

If you've got a particularly powerful car or a new car they do seem to run away with you.

Other comments related to the persuasion process itself, showing that our audience were well aware of the possible gap between good intentions and good behaviour, and illustrating the importance of targeting persuasive messages at those who would benefit most from them:

I'm not sure if it would have a long-term effect on you, but straight after you're watching it, you know, you'd start thinking about it a bit more.

I think half the time people who aren't like that do take notice and the people who are like that say, well that's not me. It just goes right through them, they can't see it at all.

In summary, both the cognitive responses and the less formal focus group discussions indicated that the overall messages of the videos were hitting home. The quantitative assessment provided a more direct test of the effectiveness of the videos on the specific beliefs targeted.

3.3 Quantitative results

After viewing the videos, participants in the quantitative assessment went on to complete the questionnaire, which contained two questions measuring each of the TPB constructs featured in the videos, together with an item measuring behavioural intention. The questionnaire also contained a previously standardized 40-item measure of general attitude to driving violations,

Table 8.2   Attitude to speeding by type of video seen

	Normative belief	Behavioural belief	Perceived behavioural control	Anticipated regret	Control
Mean	21.58	20.88	21.47	23.49	19.73
(SD)	(6.02)	(4.95)	(6.13)	(6.49)	(5.95)

the Driver Attitude Questionnaire (DAQ), which includes 10 items on attitude to speeding. A control group of drivers was used to provide baseline measures of attitudes for comparison purposes. These drivers watched an irrelevant video of similar length and style to the experimental films, featuring the same principal actor.

The key measure of the effectiveness of the videos was the comparison between the mean attitude to speeding after viewing the control video and the mean attitude to speeding after viewing each of the four experimental videos. Attitude to speeding was measured by the speeding subscale of the DAQ. Table 8.2 shows the mean scores for each of the five videos. Higher scores reflect *more negative* attitudes to speeding – that is, more desirable attitudes from a safety point of view. The video featuring the concept of anticipated regret elicited the most negative attitudes to speeding. One-way analysis of variance revealed that attitudes to speeding varied significantly as a function of video seen, $F(4, 232) = 2.56$, $p < 0.05$. Post-hoc comparisons using the Scheffé test revealed that the only statistically significant comparison was that between the control group mean and the anticipated regret group mean, $t(204) = 2.74$, $p < 0.01$.

Other findings were generally consistent with this result. As well as attitudes to speeding, *intention to speed* in the future was assessed by asking participants how likely it was that an occasion would arise during the next 12 months when they would drive down a 30 m.p.h. residential street at 40 m.p.h. They answered on a seven-point scale ranging from 'Very unlikely' to 'Very likely'. Not surprisingly, most respondents thought that they were

Table 8.3   Intention to speed by type of video seen

	Normative belief	Behavioural belief	Perceived behavioural control	Anticipated regret	Control
Mean	4.96	4.71	5.02	5.04	5.18
(SD)	(1.94)	(2.03)	(1.99)	(1.89)	(2.06)

Table 8.4 Means (and standard deviations) on TPB items by type of video seen

Item	Normative belief	Behavioural belief	Perceived behavioural control	Anticipated regret	Control	Scheffé Contrast (t)
			Type of video seen			
NB1	5.11	4.91	4.29	4.74	4.32	2.10*
	(1.45)	(1.58)	(1.62)	(1.55)	(1.61)	
NB2	5.84	5.28	5.21	5.04	4.98	2.72**
	(1.43)	(1.73)	(1.50)	(1.65)	(1.63)	
BB1	3.64	3.29	3.44	3.52	3.64	−0.83
	(2.14)	(1.91)	(1.99)	(2.06)	(1.79)	
BB2	5.38	5.27	5.54	5.38	5.10	−0.31
	(1.71)	(1.71)	(1.71)	(1.56)	(1.46)	
PBC1	5.24	4.42	3.96	4.46	4.26	−2.77**
	(1.46)	(1.63)	(1.82)	(1.68)	(1.63)	
PBC2	3.84	3.36	3.75	3.40	3.02	1.12
	(1.95)	(1.92)	(2.12)	(1.74)	(1.79)	
AR1	4.42	4.36	4.19	4.40	4.24	0.32
	(1.91)	(1.98)	(1.93)	(1.94)	(1.82)	
AR2	5.93	5.33	5.52	6.20	5.22	3.34***
	(1.36)	(1.33)	(1.47)	(1.03)	(1.36)	

Notes: *$p < 0.05$ **$p < 0.01$ ***$p < 0.001$

quite likely to speed on such a street during the next 12 months, with an overall mean of 4.99 on a seven-point scale. Table 8.3 shows that all four experimental groups had lower scores on this measure than did the control group, although the statistical comparisons between these pairs of means did not reach significance.

In addition to the measures of intention and attitudes to speeding derived from the DAQ, the questionnaire included items derived from the TPB which assessed certain aspects of our respondents' beliefs, in an effort to establish whether the videos were successful in changing the *specific* beliefs they were designed to influence. Table 8.4 shows the mean scores on these TPB items by video seen. In analysing these data, post-hoc contrasts were made to compare the TPB score for the group who had seen the relevant video with the score of participants in all other groups. It was found that those who had seen the normative beliefs video had higher scores on both of the specific beliefs targeted than participants in the other groups, reflecting the fact that they *disagreed* more with the statements that 'My partner would expect me to drive down this sort of road at 40 m.p.h.' and 'My friends would expect me to drive down this sort of road at 40 m.p.h.'

In relation to the behavioural beliefs video, the relevant items concerned the perceived likelihood of two consequences of driving down the target street at 40 m.p.h.: getting stopped by the police and putting the lives of pedestrians at risk. No significant differences were revealed by the post-hoc contrast between the group means on these items.

There was no effect of having watched the perceived behavioural control video on the perceived ease of keeping to the limit with a car on your tail. However, in relation to the perceived ease of keeping to a 30 m.p.h. limit, those who saw the PBC video had the *lowest* score, indicating that they reported that it would be neither easy nor difficult to keep to the limit in those circumstances. With the benefit of hindsight, it seems that the video, which showed someone having trouble keeping to the 30 m.p.h. limit, and being pressed quite hard by the car behind, had an effect opposite to that intended. If anything, it seemed to make viewers feel that it would be difficult to keep to the limit, when it was intended to make them think that it is important to try to exercise control over impulses to speed and to resist pressure from behind.

In relation to the anticipated regret video, the two relevant items were 'I would feel sorry for driving at 40 m.p.h. down this sort of road' and 'Driving at 40 m.p.h. down this sort of road would make me feel good' (reverse scored). For both items, the means of those who had seen the anticipated regret video tended to be higher (that is, in the predicted direction). For the 'feel good' item, the comparison was highly significant.

4 Discussion: implications for theory, policy and practice

The intervention study was designed to assess the persuasive potential of short videos, the content of which was informed by earlier empirical work identifying the beliefs that distinguished those reporting strong intentions to refrain from committing driving violations from those with relatively weak intentions. The videos featuring the concepts of *normative beliefs* and *anticipated regret* seemed to have genuine potential to improve attitudes to speeding at 40 m.p.h. in a 30 m.p.h. zone. As intended, the normative beliefs video led viewers to re-evaluate their perceptions of the wishes of their close friends and partners. The anticipated regret video was also effective in that those who saw it agreed more than other groups that speeding does not make you feel good, and expressed more negative general attitudes to speeding. Although it was difficult to operationalize the concept of anticipated regret visually, the relative success of the video provides more evidence that the concept is a valuable addition to the TPB model, at least where behaviour of some moral or personal import to the perpetrator is concerned (cf. Parker *et al.* 1995). However, further empirical work is necessary before we can be confident about the concept's potential for changing attitudes.

The *PBC* video also had a significant impact, in that those who saw it indicated the most difficulty in keeping to a 30 m.p.h. limit. Their group mean score of 3.96 shows that they felt that it would be 'neither easy nor difficult' to keep to the speed limit. If anything, the video appears to have inadvertently offered viewers a ready-made justification for speeding. The *behavioural beliefs* video, in contrast, produced no significant effect on attitudes to speeding, either generally or on TPB-specific items. One possible explanation is that suggesting that a driver might face three potential hazards on a short journey down a single residential road may have seemed unrealistic to the viewers, and caused them to discount the overall message.

The fact that the videos had no significant effect on viewers' *behavioural intentions* is unfortunate, although demonstrable and lasting attitude change is notoriously difficult to achieve (Cook and Flay 1978). In this case, the target behaviour may be especially resistant as speeding on 30 m.p.h. roads is extremely prevalent. Consequently, changing attitudes to speeding is likely to be one of the most difficult tasks facing those involved in road safety education. The inexpensive production of the videos may also have been responsible in part, as suggested by the negative comments of some viewers on technical and dramatic aspects of the videos. Drivers are part of a visually sophisticated public and are likely to criticize video material falling short of professional broadcast standards.

It is also true that the drivers who participated in this study were exposed to the persuasive attempt only twice before completing the questionnaire. A public media campaign designed to modify speeding behaviour would include repeated presentations of the persuasive communication. The role of health education in changing health behaviour is subtle and indirect. For example, in the domain of driver behaviour, campaigns encouraging the voluntary use of seat-belts were largely unsuccessful in changing behaviour (Cliff *et al.* 1980). Nevertheless, when wearing seat-belts became a legal requirement, compliance rates increased dramatically straight away. The extensive publicity given to the beneficial effects of wearing a seat-belt appears to have prepared the public to accept legislation that would otherwise have been unpopular, paving the way for an immediate change in behaviour on the introduction of legislation.

The videos may also have brought about changes not measurable by conventional attitude scales. Thus, viewing a video about speeding in a residential area may not result in immediate change of attitude but may lead people, in Prochaska and DiClemente's (1982) terms, from the 'pre-contemplative' to the 'contemplative' stage, in which they at least are considering that their behaviour might be problematic.

It is not suggested that a video-based campaign alone would be effective in changing attitudes to speeding. Rather, to be effective it is likely that videos such as these would need to be shown repeatedly, in the context of a large-scale campaign involving other forms of education, such as advertising in the print media, and higher-profile enforcement tactics. The long campaign to change drink-driving attitudes and behaviours illustrates the considerable time and effort needed. We remain convinced that the most efficient way to develop persuasive communications to influence such attitudes is to pursue the strategy of first identifying the key determinants of speeding and then trying to attack those determinants. Although our videos were produced inexpensively, we are encouraged that the evidence suggests that even two brief showings of just one is sufficient to induce more negative attitudes to speeding.

References

Ajzen, I. (1985) From intentions to actions: a theory of planned behaviour, in J. Kuhl and J. Beckman (eds) *Action Control: From Cognition to Behaviour*. Heidelberg: Springer.

Ajzen, I. and Fishbein, M. (eds) (1980) *Understanding Attitudes and Predicting Social Behavior*. Englewood Cliffs, NJ: Prentice-Hall.

Beale, D.A. and Manstead, A.S.R. (1991) Predicting mothers' intentions to limit frequency of infants' sugar intake: testing the theory of planned behavior, *Journal of Applied Social Psychology*, 21: 409–31.

Boyd, B. and Wandersman, A. (1991) Predicting undergraduate condom use with the Fishbein and Ajzen and the Triandis Attitude-Behaviour models: implications for public health interventions, *Journal of Applied Social Psychology*, 21(22): 1810–30.

Brubaker, R.G. and Fowler, C. (1990) Encouraging college males to perform testicular self-examination: evaluation of a persuasive message based on the revised theory of reasoned action, *Journal of Applied Social Psychology*, 17: 1411–22.

Budd, R.J. (1986) Predicting cigarette use: the need to incorporate measures of salience in the Theory of Reasoned Action, *Journal of Applied Social Psychology*, 16(8): 663–85.

Budd, R.J., North, D. and Spencer, C. (1984) Understanding seat-belt use: a test of Bentler and Speckart's extension of the 'theory of reasoned action', *European Journal of Social Psychology*, 14: 69–78.

Casey, S.M. and Lund, A.K. (1993) The effects of mobile roadside speedometers on traffic speeds, *Accident Analysis and Prevention*, 25: 627–34.

Cliff, K.S., Catford, J., Dillow, I. and Swann, C. (1980) Promoting the use of seat belts, *British Medical Journal*, 381: 1477–8.

Conner, M. and Sparks, P. (1996) The theory of planned behaviour and health behaviours, in M. Conner and P. Norman (eds) *Predicting Health Behaviour: Research and Practice with Social Cognition Models*. Buckingham: Open University Press.

Cook, T.D. and Flay, B.R. (1978) The persistence of experimentally induced attitude change, in L. Berkowitz (ed.) *Advances in Experimental Social Psychology*, 11. San Diego, CA: Academic Press.

Cooper, P.J. (1997) The relationship between speeding behaviour (as measured by violation convictions) and crash involvement, *Journal of Safety Research*, 28: 83–95.

Corbett, C. (1995) Road traffic offending and the introduction of speed cameras in England: the first self-report survey, *Accident Analysis and Prevention*, 27: 345–54.

Corbett, C. and Simon, F. (1992) *Unlawful Driving Behaviour: A Criminological Perspective*, contractor report no. 301. Crowthorne: Transport Research Laboratory.

Department of the Environment, Transport and the Regions (DETR) (1999) *Road Accidents Great Britain: The Casualty Report*. London: The Stationery Office.

de Waard, D. and Rooijers, T. (1994) An experimental study to evaluate the effectiveness of different methods and intensities of law enforcement on driving speed on motorways, *Accident Analysis and Prevention*, 26: 751–65.

Fishbein, M. and Ajzen, I. (1975) *Belief, Attitude, Intention and Behavior: An Introduction to Theory and Research*. Reading, MA: Addison-Wesley.

Gorsuch, R.L. and Ortberg, J. (1983) Moral obligation and attitudes: their relation to behavioural intentions, *Journal of Personality and Social Psychology*, 44(5): 1025–8.

Grube, J.W., Morgan, M. and McGree, S.T. (1986) Attitudes and normative beliefs as predictors of smoking intentions and behaviours: a test of three models, *British Journal of Social Psychology*, 25: 81–93.

Holland, C.A. and Conner, M.T. (1996) Exceeding the speed limit: an evaluation of the effectiveness of a police intervention, *Accident Analysis and Prevention*, 28: 587–97.

Kilty, K.M. (1978) Attitudinal and normative variables as predictors of drinking behavior, *Journal of Studies on Alcohol*, 39: 1178–94.

McCaul, K.D., O'Neill, H.K. and Glasgow, R.E. (1988) Predicting the performance of dental hygiene behaviours: an examination of the Fishbein and Ajzen model and self-efficacy expectations, *Journal of Applied Social Psychology*, 18(2): 114–28.

Manstead, A.S.R., Proffitt, C. and Smart, J.L. (1983) Predicting and understanding mothers' infant-feeding intentions and behaviour: testing the Theory of Reasoned Action, *Journal of Personality and Social Psychology*, 44(4): 657–71.

PACTS (1999) *Road Traffic Law and Enforcement: A Driving Force for Casualty Reduction*. London: PACTS.

Parker, D., Manstead, A.S.R., Stradling, S.G., Reason, J.T. and Baxter, J.S. (1992) Intention to commit driving violations: an application of the theory of planned behaviour, *Journal of Applied Psychology*, 77: 94–101.

Parker, D., Manstead, A.S.R. and Stradling, S.G. (1995) The role of personal norm in intentions to violate, *British Journal of Social Psychology*, 34: 127–37.

Pomazal, R.J. and Jaccard, J.J. (1976) An informational approach to altruistic behavior, *Journal of Personality and Social Psychology*, 33: 317–26.

Prochaska, J.O. and DiClemente, C.C. (1982) Transtheoretical therapy: toward a more integrative model of change, *Psychotherapy: Theory, Research and Practice*, 19: 276–88.

Richard, R., van der Pligt, J. and de Vries, N. (1996) The impact of anticipated affect on (risky) sexual behaviour, *British Journal of Social Psychology*, 34: 9–21.

Ronis, D.L. and Kaiser, M.K. (1989) Correlates of breast self-examination in a sample of college women: analyses of linear structural relations, *Journal of Applied Social Psychology*, 19: 1068–84.

Sabey, B.E. and Staughton, G.C. (1975) *The Drinking Road User in Great Britain*, supplementary report no. SR616. Crowthorne: Transport and Road Research Laboratory.

Schlegel, R.P., Crawford, C.A. and Sanborn, M.D. (1977) Correspondence and mediational properties of the Fishbein model: an application to adolescent alcohol use, *Journal of Experimental Social Psychology*, 13: 421–30.

Schnuell, R. and Lange, J. (1992) Speed reduction on through roads in Nordheim-Westfalen, *Accident Analysis and Prevention*, 24: 67–74.

Schwartz, S.H. and Tessler, R.C. (1972) A test of a model for reducing attitude-behavior inconsistencies, *Journal of Personality and Social Psychology*, 24: 225–36.

System Three (1997) *The Deterrent Effect of Enforcement in Road Safety*. Edinburgh: Scottish Central Office Research Unit.

Teed, N., Lund, A.K. and Knoblauch, R. (1993) The duration of speed reduction attributable to radar detectors, *Accident Analysis and Prevention*, 25: 131–7.

Terry, D.J., Gallois, C. and McCamish, M. (1993) *The Theory of Reasoned Action: Its Application to AIDS-related Behavior*. Oxford: Pergamon.

Vaa, T. (1997) Increased police enforcement: effects on speed, *Accident Analysis and Prevention*, 29: 373–85.

Zaidel, D., Hakkert, A.S. and Pistiner, A.H. (1992) The use of road humps for moderating speeds on urban streets, *Accident Analysis and Prevention*, 24: 45–56.

Zlatoper, T.J. (1991) Determinants of motor vehicle deaths in the United States: a cross-sectional analysis, *Accident Analysis and Prevention*, 23: 431–6.

Zuckerman, M. and Reis, H. (1978) Comparison of three models for predicting altruistic behavior, *Journal of Personality and Social Psychology*, 36: 498–510.

9 | DAPHNE EVANS AND
PAUL NORMAN

IMPROVING PEDESTRIAN ROAD SAFETY AMONG ADOLESCENTS: AN APPLICATION OF THE THEORY OF PLANNED BEHAVIOUR

This chapter considers the utility of the Theory of Planned Behaviour for informing the development of interventions to increase road safety awareness among adolescent pedestrians. The chapter begins with an overview of accident data which highlights the increased vulnerability of this age group. During adolescence it is likely that motivational and behavioural factors play an important role in accident involvement. A survey of over 1800 school children (Evans 1999) employed the TPB to examine the motivational determinants of potentially hazardous road-crossing decisions. On the basis of the results of this survey, a school drama group (n = 13) was invited to devise and develop a short theatre intervention to increase road safety awareness among adolescent pedestrians. The theatre piece was then performed to a group of school children (n = 88) who completed TPB questionnaires two weeks before the performance and again directly afterwards. A control group (n = 141) completed the questionnaires on two occasions separated by two weeks. After watching the theatre piece, the school children reported more negative behavioural and normative beliefs. In contrast, the beliefs of the control group remained stable over time. In addition, pupils in the drama group, who completed TPB questionnaires before and after developing the theatre piece, reported more negative intentions and lower perceptions of control about crossing the road in a potentially hazardous manner at the end of the project. The results are discussed in relation to the potential of school-based theatre interventions to increase road safety awareness and the need to engage recipients of the intervention actively so that they process the road safety information being presented systematically.

1 Improving pedestrian road safety among adolescents

1.1 Incidence and characteristics of pedestrian accidents

In 1998, over 17,000 children were killed or injured in pedestrian accidents (DETR 1999), which represent 'the single, biggest accidental killer of children and adolescents in Britain' (Avery and Jackson 1993). Ward *et al.* (1994) report that 10–15-year-olds have the highest casualty rates per 100,000 of the population, per 100 million pedestrian kilometres walked and per 100 million roads crossed. As a result, one child in fifteen is injured in a road traffic accident before his or her sixteenth birthday (Jones 1990).

While accident statistics have reduced in recent years, the absolute number of pedestrian casualties among children remains high. Moreover, it is likely that this reduction is not due to road safety education, but rather to decreased pedestrian exposure. Roberts (1993) reports that child pedestrian casualty rates have fallen as car ownership has increased. Thus, for example, as children are increasingly being transported to school by car their exposure to risk is decreasing. However, this is related to socio-economic status as car ownership is lower among lower income families. This, in part, may account for the finding that children from the lowest socio-economic group are four times more likely to die through pedestrian injury than those from the highest socio-economic group (Christie 1995). In addition, children from lower socio-economic backgrounds play in the street more frequently, which further increases their pedestrian risk.

A comprehensive review of road safety research by Tight (1996) reveals a number of common features in child pedestrian casualties. First, it has been found that child pedestrian accidents typically peak between 8 and 9 a.m. and again between 3 and 6 p.m. (Tight 1987). These times coincide with the journey to and from school, supporting Grayson's (1975) observation that 50 per cent of accidents occur between 4 and 5 p.m. during school term time. Second, the majority of the accidents occur on urban roads (Southwell *et al.* 1990) and within a quarter of a mile of the child's home (Grayson 1975). Third, boys are twice as likely as girls to be involved in a pedestrian accident (Pless *et al.* 1989), perhaps because they are more likely to play in the road. Fourth, involvement in pedestrian accidents peaks around 12 years of age. This coincides with entry into secondary education, a time when children are often afforded greater freedom of movement (Lynam and Harland 1992). Finally, a number of studies have found that the majority of accidents occur when the child is intent on crossing the road (Grayson 1975; Southwell *et al.* 1990). Moreover, these studies have demonstrated that children typically engage in three risky pre-crossing activities. First, they will often fail to stop at the kerb. Second, they will often fail to check that the road is clear before crossing. Third, they are often running and, although stopping momentarily at the kerb, pay little attention to the traffic environment.

In addition, research has revealed a number of perceptual errors made by children when crossing the road (Tight *et al.* 1990). For example, when looking at oncoming vehicles, children often make cognitive errors arising from misjudgements of speed and/or distance.

1.2 Previous research on pedestrian accidents

In addition to the research outlined above that has examined the character-istics of pedestrian accidents, studies of the causes of accident involvement among children have focused on the development of perceptual skills and 'risk-taking' behaviour. A number have found that young children do not have the perceptual or cognitive skills that are required to cross the road safely (Avery and Jackson 1993; Demetre and Gaffin 1994). For example, in a study by Whitebread and Neilson (1996) groups of children aged 4–11 years were given a series of tasks to test their pedestrian skills. In one of the tasks the children were shown a set of twelve slides of road-crossing scenarios and were asked to indicate a safe place to cross. In another task the children were shown a video of oncoming traffic, which was frozen at various points, and were asked to indicate whether it was safe to cross. Whitebread and Neilson (1996) found that young children had little or no understanding of what constitutes a safe place to cross and were poor at making judgements about crossing in sight of oncoming traffic. However, Whitebread and Neilson (1996) also concluded that the majority of older children (that is, adolescents) had acquired the skills necessary to cross the road safely. This implies that, among adolescents, it is not the failure to acquire adequate road-crossing skills, but the failure to employ these skills that may be the major determinant of accident involvement. For example, Tight *et al.* (1990) have identified three principal reasons for the failure of adolescents to employ these skills: distraction from the task, hurriedness, and thoughtlessness.

A number of researchers have identified a link between antisocial behavi-our and/or delinquency and children's proneness to accidents in general (Bijur and Stewart-Brown 1986; Wadsworth 1987; Junger *et al.* 1995; Thuen and Bendixen 1996) and road traffic accidents in particular (Pless *et al.* 1989; West and Farr 1989). It may be the case that some individuals have a predisposition, or personality trait, that influences their behaviour and makes them more prone to accidents. Zuckerman *et al.* (1978), for example, argue for the existence of such a sensation-seeking personality trait, and have reported evidence linking sensation seeking with a range of maladaptive or risky behaviours such as greater sexual activity, drug use, smoking and participation in physically dangerous activities. In addition, children identi-fied as having conduct behaviour problems and attending special clinics have also been found to have elevated sensation-seeking scores (Russo *et al.* 1993). Nevertheless, as West *et al.* (1999) suggest, there are likely to be further motivational factors that account for the increased proneness of adolescents to pedestrian accidents.

1.3 Road safety education

Road safety education is often provided to children from an early age. For example, in many parts of the UK, there are 'Children's Traffic Clubs', which children are invited to join on their third birthday. If parents take up this option, the children are sent simple road safety information at six-monthly intervals. Parents are encouraged to work through the material with their child to raise awareness of road safety. Where the scheme is used wholeheartedly, it has been found to be an effective introduction to road safety education for pre-school children. For young children (that is, 5–11-year-olds), many local authorities adopt 'Further Ahead' – a package developed by the Royal Society for the Prevention of Accidents to be used in conjunction with the key stages in the national school curriculum. However, the provision of road safety education in schools is not uniform. Moreover, learning road safety in a classroom environment may lead to the material being learned more as theoretical concepts than as practical skills. As a result, there has been a recent trend towards the development of practical pedestrian skills training for young children (Thomson *et al.* 1996).

The provision of road safety education among 11–15-year-olds in secondary schools is sparse. Research by Singh and Spear (1989) found that only a minority of secondary schools have any road safety education provision, despite the fact that a substantial number of pedestrian accidents in this age group occur on journeys to and from school. In addition, it is likely that road safety education for this age group will need to focus on different factors from those selected at primary school. It is clear that, by the age of 11, the vast majority of children have already acquired the cognitive and perceptual skills to cross the road safely. Thus, it may be the failure to deploy these skills that contributes to the high rate of pedestrian casualties among adolescents. As a result, interventions that focus on the motivational determinants of unsafe road-crossing behaviour may be more efficacious.

2 Theoretical perspective: the Theory of Planned Behaviour

2.1 Intervening through the TPB

Previous work has shown that the majority of child pedestrian accidents occur when the child is going to or from school (Tight 1996) and is intent on crossing the road (Southwell *et al.* 1990). In addition, most pedestrian accidents occur when the child attempts to cross the road away from a designated crossing point (Avery and Jackson 1993). Thus, a clearer understanding of the motivational determinants of 'risky' decisions is likely to aid the development of road safety interventions aimed at the 11–15-year-old age group.

One model that might be usefully employed in this context is the Theory of Planned Behaviour (Ajzen 1988, 1991). As we have seen in earlier chapters, the TPB has been applied successfully to a range of social and health behaviours (see Conner and Sparks 1996; Armitage and Conner 1998), with meta-analyses revealing that the TPB typically explains between 40 and 50 per cent of the variance in behavioural intention (Sutton 1998). One of the attractions of the TPB is its relative parsimony; that is, it provides a simple model of the proximal determinants of individuals' decisions (that is, intentions). However, a number of researchers have argued that the predictive power of the model may be improved through the inclusion of additional variables. Three such variables may be relevant in the present context. First, a distinction can be made between subjective norms (that is, the perception of social pressure to perform a behaviour) and personal or moral norms (that is, the individual's perception of the moral correctness or incorrectness of performing the behaviour) (Ajzen 1991; Manstead 2000). Thus, moral norms that take account of 'personal feelings of . . . responsibility to perform, or refuse to perform, a certain behavior' (Ajzen 1991: 199) may be a further, independent, form of normative pressure. Armitage and Conner (1998), in their review of the TPB, report that the addition of moral norms typically produces a small, but significant, increment in the amount of variance explained in intention. Second, anticipated feelings associated with the performance of the behaviour may also be an important determinant of an individual's decision to perform a behaviour (Triandis 1977). Recent research has focused on the influence of anticipated regret, finding that those individuals who anticipate feeling regret after performing a behaviour are less likely to intend to perform the behaviour (for example Richard *et al.* 1996). However, in the present context it is likely that individuals may also expect to experience positive emotions following 'risky' road-crossing behaviours, which may influence their decisions. Third, self-identity (that is, the labels individuals use to describe themselves) may also predict intentions to perform a behaviour (Biddle *et al.* 1987; Charng *et al.* 1988). For example, Sparks and Shepherd (1992) found that individuals who saw themselves as 'green consumers' were more likely to intend to consume organic vegetables. This effect was over and above the influence of the TPB variables. In the present context, the extent to which individuals see themselves as 'safe pedestrians' may influence their road-crossing behaviour.

The TRA and the TPB have been applied to a range of road safety behaviours. For example, the TRA has been used to predict seat-belt use (Wittenbraker *et al.* 1983; Budd *et al.* 1984; Martin and Newman 1990; Stasson and Fishbein 1990; Thuen and Rise 1994) and the use of car seats and restraints for children (Gielen *et al.* 1984), as well as motorcycling behaviour (Rutter *et al.* 1995). The TPB has been applied to three main road user groups: drivers, cyclists and pedestrians. Parker *et al.* (1992) used the TPB to examine drivers' intentions to commit driving violations. Drivers were presented with scenarios depicting a number of common driving violations (that is, drink-driving, speeding, close following, risky overtaking) followed by items measuring the main TPB constructs. The TPB was able to explain between 23 and 47 per cent of the variance in intentions, with attitude, subjective norm and perceived behavioural control all emerging as significant independent predictors. More recently, Parker *et al.* (1995) tested an extended version of the TPB to examine intentions to commit motorway driving violations (for example overtaking on the inside). Again, all three components of the TPB were predictive of intentions, explaining between 34 and 37 per cent of the variance. However, the additional variables of moral norms and anticipated affect made significant contributions to the prediction of intentions to commit violations over and above the influence of the TPB variables. Considering cyclists, two studies have successfully applied the TPB to safety helmet use among school children (Sissons Joshi *et al.* 1994; Quine *et al.* 1998). For example, Quine *et al.* (1998) found that the TPB was able to explain 34 per cent of the variance in intentions to wear a safety helmet and 43 per cent of the variance in reported safety helmet use at one month follow-up among a sample of 11–18-year-old schoolboys. Subjective norm and perceived behavioural control were the strongest predictors of intention, with intention and perceived behavioural control predicting actual safety helmet use. Evans and Norman (1998) used a similar methodology to that used by Parker *et al.* (1992, 1995) to examine adult pedestrians' road-crossing decisions in response to three potentially hazardous road-crossing scenarios (for example crossing a busy dual carriageway). The TPB was able to explain between 37 and 49 per cent of the variance in pedestrians' intentions to cross the road in the manner depicted in the scenarios. In addition, a measure of self-identity led to small but significant increments in the amounts of variance explained in intention for two of the three scenarios.

Considering adolescents' road-crossing decisions, Evans (1999) completed a survey of over 1800 secondary school children in South Wales. Respondents were presented with two potentially hazardous road-crossing scenarios (that is, crossing a busy road, crossing from behind a bus) followed by items measuring the main TPB constructs and the additional variables of moral norms, anticipated affect and self-identity. The TPB was able to explain between 21 and 27 per cent of the variance in intentions to cross the road in the manner depicted in the two scenarios, with all three components emerging as significant predictors. The additional variables produced significant increments in the amounts of variance explained, although only anticipated affect and self-identity emerged as significant predictors. In both scenarios, attitude and self-identity were the most powerful predictors of road-crossing intentions. More detailed analysis of individual behavioural beliefs revealed that, for both scenarios, the beliefs that crossing the road in the manner depicted would be easier and would get children home more quickly were strongly correlated with intentions. For normative beliefs, the views of friends were found to have the strongest impact on intentions for both scenarios. These findings suggest three main avenues that interventions designed to encourage safer road-crossing behaviour among adolescents may explore. First, they should focus on the belief that crossing the road in a potentially dangerous manner necessarily leads to easier and quicker journeys. Second, given the importance of self-identity as a predictor, interventions should aim to increase adolescents' views of themselves as 'safe pedestrians' and encourage a more 'thoughtful' approach to road crossing. Third, interventions should take advantage of the powerful influence of friends and peers among this age group to change attitudes and behaviour.

2.2 Theatre and drama interventions

One potentially useful way of presenting a road safety message is through the use of a theatre intervention in which adolescents watch a play, usually performed by a professional theatre company, that has been designed to focus on road safety issues. Theatre interventions are likely to engage the audience and present material in ways that are easy to understand. Thus, members of the audience are likely to be motivated and have the cognitive ability to process the material contained in the intervention (Petty and Cacioppo 1986). Powney *et al.* (1995) have suggested that theatre interventions in schools have a number of advantages over other more traditional modes of presentation. In particular, they may be a useful method for dealing with sensitive social issues and are likely to have a greater 'impact', which may motivate students to consider the issues presented and thereby change their attitudes and behaviour.

A number of studies have evaluated the use of theatre interventions in schools, although they have produced mixed results. For example, Gliksman *et al.* (1984) assessed the impact of a theatrical performance focusing on alcohol use on the knowledge, attitudes and behaviour of Canadian high school students. It was found that the performance had a significant impact on attitudes and behaviour, although this impact was no greater than that of a more traditional lesson plan intervention. Powney *et al.* (1995) evaluated the impact of a theatre tour, focusing on drink-driving, in five schools in Scotland and Wales. The study compared three interventions. The first was a performance by a professional theatre group of a play detailing a true story of two sisters in an alcohol-related fatal road accident. The second was a presentation by a road safety officer based on a television documentary on drink-driving. The third was a teacher presentation of a road safety video. Following each of the presentations, the students engaged in discussion groups to explore in more detail the issues raised. The results indicated that, following the presentations, students had better knowledge and more negative attitudes towards drink-driving. However, no differences were found between the intervention groups in knowledge or attitudes, although students watching the theatre presentation reported that they found it more enjoyable, harder hitting, and more informative than the other presentations.

Given the finding reported by Evans (1999) that the views of friends have a strong influence on adolescents' road-crossing intentions, the impact of theatre interventions may be further increased by using peers to design and perform the intervention. Such an argument is consistent with research by Telch *et al.* (1990), who evaluated a peer-led smoking prevention programme in which peer teachers led a number of sessions to help younger students to develop strategies to resist social pressures to smoke cigarettes. Significant differences were found between the intervention and control groups at nine-month follow-up. Peer-led interventions may be effective for a number of reasons. First, the level of understanding between same-age participants is better. Second, there are no language barriers, because participants use and understand the same colloquial words and expressions. Third, participants are likely to be more receptive and responsive to suggestions from their peers. Thus, a road safety theatre intervention that is developed and performed by similar aged students may have the requisite characteristics to motivate and enable recipients to reconsider their attitudes towards pedestrian road safety.

In addition to having an impact on the recipients of the theatre presentation, it is likely that those responsible for developing and producing the intervention will have their views about pedestrian road safety challenged. Thus, a distinction can be made between theatre interventions, in which participants watch a theatre production, and drama interventions, in which participants work together over a period of time to produce a drama piece. The use of drama may have several benefits, including the ability to encourage exploration and illumination (O'Neill *et al.* 1989). Thus, participation in drama interventions may encourage the systematic processing of information that is likely to lead to changes in attitudes and behaviour (Heppner *et al.* 1995). For example, studies have found that participation in drama interventions can lead to increased knowledge about AIDS (Dalrymple and Du Toit 1993), increased seat-belt use (Lehman and Scott 1990) and improved interpersonal cognitive problem solving (Johnston *et al.* 1985).

3 The intervention

The development of the drama piece to be used in the theatre intervention study took place over a number of sessions in a six-week period. In the first session, the first author asked the pupils to complete a TPB questionnaire on road crossing (see below) and then introduced the topic of road safety to the group. The pupils were informed of the broad aims of the project (that is, research into the road crossing behaviour of 11–15-year-olds). In addition, figures on the number of young people killed or injured in pedestrian road accidents each year were supplied. Finally, a summary of the results from the survey of adolescents' road safety attitudes (Evans 1999) was presented, which emphasized the importance of attitudes, self-identity and friends' beliefs on road-crossing decisions. With the help of their drama teacher, the group was then invited to produce a 15-minute play based on the information given. It was emphasized that the information should be interpreted in their own style, using whatever topical information they thought might reinforce the road safety message. Before the second session, the pupils were asked to observe their own and their peers' road-crossing behaviour. In the next session, these observations were discussed in light of what the group might already know about safe road crossing (that is, the Green Cross Code) and the information presented in the first session. The group then developed their drama piece over the next few weeks and finally performed it in front of invited audiences.

3.1 Participants and procedure

Theatre intervention
Two schools agreed to take part in the study, and the pupils from Year 7 (11–12 years old) in each school were allocated to either the 'theatre' condition or the control condition. Each school was visited twice. During the first visit the first author introduced the broad aims of the research and the pupils completed the TPB questionnaire. In the second visit to the theatre condition school, pupils in Year 7 (n = 88) saw a live performance of the intervention developed by the drama group and then completed the TPB for a second time. In the control condition school, pupils in the same year (n = 141) completed the TPB for a second time before watching a live performance of the intervention.

Drama intervention
Thirteen pupils in a Year 11 (15–16 years old) drama group were invited to participate in the development and production of a road safety intervention. The drama project took place over six weeks and pupils completed the TPB questionnaire at the start of the project and again at the end.

Questionnaire
The questionnaire described a potentially dangerous road-crossing behaviour. The scenario was written in the second person singular in order to encourage respondents to imagine themselves in it. The scenario was as follows:

You are on your way home from school. It is cold, so you are hurrying home. About half-way from home, you have to cross a busy road – there is a crossing further down the road, but that will take you a lot longer to get home because you will then have to walk back up the other side. You cannot see any vehicles coming so you run across the road.

The respondents were then asked to answer a series of questions, based on the TPB, about the scenario. All items were followed by seven-point response scales, with descriptive labels to aid comprehension and understanding. *Behavioural intention* was measured using two items. Respondents were asked to indicate how likely it was that they would run across the road, first if they were the person in the description, and second, if they came across a similar situation themselves in the next few weeks (scored −3 to +3). The mean of the two items was used as a measure of behavioural intention. This measure was found to have satisfactory internal reliability at Time 1 and Time 2 (alphas = 0.79, 0.80). Respondents' *attitude* towards crossing the road as depicted in the scenario was measured using four semantic differential scales (for example 'Running across the road, as described, would be . . . bad/good') (scored −3 to +3). The mean of the four items was used as a measure of attitude (alphas = 0.84, 0.88). *Subjective norm* was measured using a single item ('Most people who are important to me would think that I should run across the road') (scored −3 to +3). Three items were used to measure *perceived behavioural control*, but subsequent analyses revealed that they did not form a reliable scale. As a result, only one item, asking how difficult or easy it would be to cross the road, was used as a measured of perceived behavioural control ('If I were the person in this description, I think running across the road would be . . . difficult/easy') (scored −3 to +3).

A number of additional variables were measured in the questionnaire. *Moral norms* were measured using two items. Respondents were asked to indicate the extent to which they felt they ought not to cross the road as described in the scenario (for example 'I shouldn't really run across the road') (scored −3 to +3). The mean of the two items was used as a measure of moral norms and was found to have satisfactory internal reliability at both time points (alphas = 0.67, 0.61). *Anticipated affect* was measured using two items that focused on respondents' feelings about running across the road (for example 'Running across the road would make me feel big') (scored −3 to +3). The mean of the two items was used as a measure of anticipated affect (alphas = 0.77, 0.75). Finally, in order to measure *self-identity*, respondents were asked two more general questions about their view of themselves as safe pedestrians (for example 'I like to think of myself as a careful pedestrian') (scored −3 to +3). The mean of the two items was used as a measure of self-identity (alphas = 0.72, 0.80).

In addition to the direct measures outlined above, the questionnaire also measured behavioural beliefs and normative beliefs towards the behaviour depicted in the scenario. The modal salient beliefs for the scenario were generated through pilot interviews with 61 children, following the recommendations of Ajzen and Fishbein (1980). Control beliefs were not measured, as the pilot interviews revealed a large overlap with the modal salient behavioural beliefs. Four *behavioural beliefs* were used in the questionnaire. Belief strength (for example 'Running across the road, as described, could get me run over') was assessed using a response scale ranging from 'Very unlikely' (−3) to 'Very likely' (+3). For each belief statement there was a corresponding outcome evaluation (for example 'Getting run over would be . . . very bad/very good') (scored −3 to +3). The products of the pairs of items were averaged to provide a summary measure of behavioural beliefs. Four referents were used to measure *normative beliefs*. Respondents were asked to indicate whether each referent would approve of them crossing the road in the manner depicted (for example 'My friends would think I should run across the road') (scored −3 to +3) and the extent to which they were motivated to comply with their views (for example 'I generally like to cross the road in a way that my friends think I should') (scored −3 to +3). The products of the pairs of items were averaged to provide a summary measure of normative beliefs.

3.2 Results

Theatre intervention

A MANOVA was performed to examine the effect of the experimental conditions (theatre/control) over time (Time 1/Time 2) on the dependent variables. Overall, the main effect of condition was found to be non-significant (F = 1.83, df = 9,186, NS). However, the main effect of time (F = 3.19, df = 9,186, p < 0.01) and the condition × time interaction (F = 2.79, df = 9,186, p < 0.01) were both found to be significant. The F values from the univariate analyses for the main effects of condition and time and the condition × time interaction are presented in Table 9.1, and the means of each variable for each condition over time are presented in Table 9.2.

As shown in Table 9.1, significant univariate effects were found for only two variables, behavioural beliefs and normative beliefs. For behavioural beliefs, the main effects of condition and time, as well as the interaction between condition and time, were all found to be significant. Inspection of the means in Table 9.2 reveals that respondents in the theatre condition had more negative behavioural belief scores than those in the control condition, and that over time behavioural belief scores became more negative. Post-hoc analysis of the interaction revealed that while the behavioural belief scores of the control condition remained relatively stable between Time 1

Table 9.1   Theatre intervention: univariate ANOVA summary table (F values)

Variable	Condition	Time	Condition × time
Intention	1.60	3.53	1.78
Attitude	1.38	0.01	0.02
Subjective norm	0.63	0.69	2.64
Perceived behavioural control	1.06	0.38	0.14
Moral norms	0.02	0.04	2.15
Anticipated affect	0.01	1.64	1.49
Self-identity	0.48	1.14	1.95
Behavioural beliefs	6.89*	9.07**	7.40*
Normative beliefs	3.17	7.15**	8.38**

Notes: * $p < 0.05$ ** $p < 0.01$

Table 9.2   Theatre intervention: means of the variables under consideration by condition (control/theatre) and time

Variable	Time 1		Time 2	
	Control	Theatre	Control	Theatre
Intention	−0.75	−1.22	−0.68	−0.81
Attitude	−1.86	−2.02	−1.84	−2.02
Subjective norm	−2.46	−2.11	−2.13	−2.22
Perceived behavioural control	−0.87	−1.06	−0.71	−1.02
Moral norms	1.48	1.27	1.28	1.43
Anticipated affect	−1.70	−1.55	−1.37	−1.53
Self-identity	1.38	1.34	1.35	1.37
Behavioural beliefs	−2.26	−2.49	−2.33	−3.85
Normative beliefs	−2.26	−0.61	−2.20	−2.25

and Time 2 ($t = 0.27$, $df = 140$, NS), the scores of the theatre condition became more negative over time ($t = 3.69$, $df = 54$, $p < 0.01$). As a result, while there was no difference between the two conditions at Time 1 ($t = 0.60$, $df = 194$, NS), at Time 2 respondents in the theatre condition had more negative behavioural beliefs than those in the control condition ($t = 3.48$, $df = 194$, $p < 0.01$).

Considering normative beliefs, the main effect of time and the condition × time interaction were found to be significant. Inspection of the means in Table 9.2 reveals that between Time 1 and Time 2 scores on this measure became more negative. Post-hoc analysis of the interaction revealed that while the normative belief scores of the control condition remained relatively stable between Time 1 and Time 2 (t = 0.20, df = 140, NS), the scores of the theatre condition became more negative over time (t = 3.47, df = 54, p < 0.01). However, post-hoc analysis of the interaction also revealed that the two conditions were not equivalent at Time 1, in that respondents in the theatre condition had less negative normative beliefs than those in the control condition (t = 3.45, df = 194, p < 0.01). As a result of the reduction in normative belief scores between Time 1 and Time 2 in the theatre condition, the two conditions did not differ at Time 2 (t = 0.08, df = 194, NS).

Drama intervention
The responses of the children involved in the development of the drama piece to the evaluation questionnaire at the start and end of the project were analysed using Wilcoxon signed-ranks tests. As can be seen from Table 9.3, both intention and perceived behavioural control showed significant reductions over time. Thus, at the end of the project, the children were less likely than at the beginning to intend to run across the road as described in the scenario and were less likely to believe that doing so would be easy.

Table 9.3 Drama intervention: means of the variables under consideration over time (Wilcoxon's Z-values)

Variable	Time 1	Time 2	Z-value
Intention	1.15	−0.31	2.62**
Attitude	−1.57	−1.52	0.25
Subjective norm	−2.69	−2.46	0.80
Perceived behavioural control	0.58	−0.08	2.27*
Moral norms	1.31	1.31	0.25
Anticipated affect	−1.73	−1.73	0.51
Self-identity	0.88	1.08	0.42
Behavioural beliefs	−1.85	−1.73	0.31
Normative beliefs	−0.25	0.48	0.86

Notes: * p < 0.05   ** p < 0.01

4 Discussion: implications for theory, policy and practice

This study sought to evaluate the impact of a TPB-based theatre intervention on adolescents' pedestrian road safety attitudes. On the basis of an earlier study (Evans 1999) that had examined the motivational determinants of adolescents' road-crossing intentions, a school drama class was invited to develop a road safety theatre intervention. The intervention was then performed to a group of school children, who completed a TPB question-naire two weeks before the intervention and again directly afterwards. Another group of school children was used as a control group, completing the TPB questionnaire at two time points separated by two weeks. The results of the study indicated that the intervention had only a modest effect on the attitudes of the children who watched the intervention. None of the direct measures of the TPB constructs or the additional variables under consideration were found to have changed as a result of the intervention in comparison with the control condition. However, significant effects were found for behavioural beliefs and normative beliefs, in that the beliefs of children who watched the theatre intervention became more negative over time while the beliefs of children in the control group remained stable. Thus, after watching the intervention, the children were less likely to believe that running across the road as depicted in the scenario would lead to positive outcomes and less likely to believe that it would attract social approval.

While the intervention was designed to capture the recipients' attention and thereby encourage the active processing of the content, it is clear from the results that the intervention had only a relatively modest impact on road safety attitudes. Moreover, given that the theatre intervention was compared only with a no-intervention control condition, we cannot be sure that its impact on behavioural and normative beliefs was any greater than that of more traditional road safety education lessons. Powney *et al.* (1995) like-wise reported that a theatre intervention on drink-driving attitudes was no more effective than a presentation led by a road safety officer or teacher, and similar results have been reported by Gliksman *et al.* (1984) in relation to alcohol use.

There are a number of possible reasons for the relatively modest impact of the theatre intervention in the present study. First, the intervention was very brief, lasting only 15 minutes. It may be necessary to design more intensive interventions to produce stronger changes in road safety attitudes and behaviour. For example, further follow-up discussion groups may be required, to explore the issues raised by the intervention in more detail (Powney *et al.* 1995). Second, the school children completed the second TPB questionnaire directly after watching the intervention. It may be the case that they did not have the opportunity to consider or process the content of the intervention fully. Third, while school children may enjoy watching a theatre intervention, this does not necessarily lead to a differential impact over other road safety education methods (Powney *et al.* 1995). Fourth, while the presentation of the theatre intervention by similarly aged peers may increase the salience of the message, the influence of peers on attitudes and behaviour may be limited to close friends and associates (Blyth *et al.* 1982). The above points suggest that watching a theatre intervention may, in itself, not be sufficient to encourage the systematic processing of in-formation that is crucial for changes in attitudes and behaviour (Petty and

Cacioppo 1986). Watching a theatre intervention may be a passive, rather than an active, experience. Such interventions may need to be followed up with additional sessions to explore the issues raised in the intervention in more detail. However, as Powney *et al.* (1995) note in their evaluation of theatre interventions in schools, follow-up work is often not carried out, because of timetable pressures from examined subjects.

An alternative approach is to use the development of the theatre piece as an intervention in itself. In the present study a school drama class was invited to develop the intervention as a class project over a six-week period. Their responses to the TPB questionnaire completed at the beginning and end of the project indicated significant reductions in intention and perceived behavioural control. Thus, at the end of the project the pupils were less likely to report that they would run across the road as depicted in the scenario and less likely to believe that doing so would be easy. While the small sample size and the lack of a control group mean that the findings should be treated with caution they are, nevertheless, encouraging. Intention and perceived behavioural control are the two proximal determinants of behaviour in the TPB; research by Parker (1997) has found that respondents' indications of their intentions in response to road safety scenarios are related to their actual observed behaviour.

The use of drama interventions has been found to stimulate exploration, illumination (O'Neill *et al.* 1989) and the use of systematic processing of material to be included in the theatre piece (Heppner *et al.* 1995). Thus, drama encourages thinking over impulsiveness. Assisting children to develop thinking skills can help to reduce impulsive or careless behaviour (Hyman 1994). This is important as a number of researchers have concluded that careless or reckless behaviour is a major cause of involvement in road traffic accidents (Elander *et al.* 1993; West *et al.* 1999). A further advantage of the use of drama interventions is that they can be incorporated into the school timetable, thus ensuring a prolonged and detailed consideration of road safety issues. Nevertheless, it still needs to be shown that the use of a drama intervention to encourage safer road safety attitudes and behaviour is more effective than other more traditional methods.

In conclusion, the work presented in this chapter has highlighted the utility of the TPB for identifying the motivational determinants of adolescents' road-crossing decisions, and has shown that the model can be used as a framework for developing a road safety intervention to target beliefs related to making unsafe road-crossing decisions. However, while the TPB can identify which beliefs to target, it does not outline how to change these beliefs. Instead it is necessary to consider theories of persuasion and attitude change that emphasize the importance of encouraging recipients to process the content of an intervention systematically (Petty and Cacioppo 1986; Eagly and Chaiken 1993). Previous work has suggested that theatre interventions may be a suitable medium through which to present road safety education to adolescents. However, the results of the present study indicated that a theatre intervention developed by a school drama class had only a relatively modest impact on road safety attitudes. To be effective, it is likely that follow-up discussion groups will be needed, to explore the issues raised by the intervention in more detail. An alternative approach is to view the development of the theatre piece as an intervention in its own right, which may encourage participants to process road safety information systematically. In this study, participation in a drama intervention was found to have an impact both on intentions and on perceptions of control. However, these initial findings will need to be replicated in future studies, with larger sample sizes and appropriate control groups. This may confirm the potential of the TPB as a framework for developing effective road safety interventions to change attitudes and behaviour, and in turn may help to reduce the number of pedestrian road traffic casualties among adolescents.

References

Ajzen, I. (1988) *Attitudes, Personality and Behavior*. Milton Keynes: Open University Press.

Ajzen, I. (1991) The Theory of Planned Behavior, *Organizational Behavior and Human Decision Processes*, 50: 179–211.

Ajzen, I. and Fishbein, M. (eds) (1980) *Understanding Attitudes and Predicting Social Behavior*. Englewood Cliffs, NJ: Prentice-Hall.

Armitage, C. and Conner, M. (1998) Extending the theory of planned behavior: a review and avenues for further research, *Journal of Applied Social Psychology*, 28: 1429–64.

Avery, J.G. and Jackson, R. (1993) *Children and their Accidents*. London: Arnold.

Biddle, B., Bank, B. and Slavings, R. (1987) Norms, preferences, identities and retention decisions, *Social Psychology Quarterly*, 50: 322–37.

Bijur, P.E. and Stewart-Brown, S. (1986) Child behavior and accidental injury in 11,966 pre-school children, *American Journal of Diseases of Children*, 40: 487–93.

Blyth, D., Hill, J. and Thiel, K. (1982) Early adolescents' significant others: grade and gender differences in perceived relationships with familial and non-familial adults and young people, *Journal of Youth and Adolescence*, 11: 425–50.

Budd, R.J., North, D. and Spencer, C. (1984) Understanding seat-belt use: a test of Bentler and Speckart's extension of the 'theory of reasoned action', *European Journal of Social Psychology*, 14: 69–78.

Charng, H.W., Piliavin, J.A. and Callero, P.L. (1988) Role identity and reasoned action in the prediction of repeated behavior, *Social Psychology Quarterly*, 51: 303–17.

Christie, N. (1995) *Social, Economic and Environmental Factors in Child Pedestrian Accidents: A Research Review*, TRRL report no. 116. London: Department of Transport.

Conner, M. and Sparks, P. (1996) The theory of planned behaviour and health behaviours, in M. Conner and P. Norman (eds) *Predicting Health Behaviour:*

Research and Practice with Social Cognition Models. Buckingham: Open University Press.

Dalrymple, L. and Du Toit, M.K. (1993) The evaluation of a drama approach to AIDS education, *Educational Psychology*, 13: 147–54.

Demetre, J.D. and Gaffin, S. (1994) The salience of occluding vehicles to child pedestrians, *British Journal of Educational Psychology*, 64: 243–51.

Department of the Environment, Transport and the Regions (DETR) (1999) *Road Accidents Great Britain: The Casualty Report*. London: The Stationery Office.

Eagly, A.H. and Chaiken, S. (1993) *The Psychology of Attitudes*. New York: Harcourt Brace and Jovanovich.

Elander, J., West, R. and French, D. (1993) Behavioural correlates of individual differences in road traffic crash risk: an examination of methods and findings, *Psychological Bulletin*, 113: 279–94.

Evans, D. (1999) Understanding and changing road safety awareness in adolescents. PhD thesis, University of Wales Swansea.

Evans, D. and Norman, P. (1998) Understanding pedestrians' road crossing decisions: an application of the theory of planned behaviour, *Health Education Research*, 13: 481–9.

Gielen, A.C., Erikson, M.P., Daltroy, L.H. and Rost, K. (1984) Factors associated with the use of child restraint devices, *Health Education Quarterly*, 11(2): 195–206.

Gliksman, L., Douglas, R.R. and Smythe, C. (1984) The impact of a high school alcohol education program utilizing a live theatrical performance: a comparative study, *Journal of Drug Education*, 13: 229–48.

Grayson, G.B. (1975) *Observations of Pedestrians at Four Sites*, Department of the Environment report no. 670. Crowthorne: Transport and Road Research Laboratory.

Heppner, M.J., Humphrey, C.F., Hillenbrand-Gunn, T.L. and DeBord, K.A. (1995) The differential effects of rape prevention programming on attitudes, behavior, and knowledge, *Journal of Counseling Psychology*, 42: 508–18.

Hyman, M.H. (1994) Impulsive behaviour: a case for helping children 'think' about change, *Educational Psychology in Practice*, 10: 141–8.

Johnston, J.C., Healey, K.N. and Tracey-Magid, D. (1985) Drama and interpersonal problem solving: a dynamic interplay for adolescent groups, *Child Care Quarterly*, 14: 238–47.

Jones, D. (1990) *Child Casualties in Road Accidents*. London: Department of Transport.

Junger, M., Terlouw, G. and van der Heijden, P. (1995) Crime, accidents and social control, *Criminal Behaviour and Mental Health*, 5: 386–410.

Lehman, G.R. and Scott, G.E. (1990) Participative education for children: an effective approach to increase safety belt use, *Journal of Applied Behavior Analysis*, 23: 219–25.

Lynam, D. and Harland, D. (1992) *Child Pedestrian Safety in the UK*. Berlin: VTI/FERSI Conference.

Manstead, A.S.R. (2000) The role of moral norm in the attitude–behavior relationship, in D.J. Terry and M.A. Hogg (eds) *Attitudes, Behavior and Social Context: The Role of Norms and Group Membership*. Mahwah, NJ: Lawrence Erlbaum.

Martin, G.L. and Newman, I.M. (1990) Women as motivators in the use of safety belts, *Health Values, Health Behavior, Education and Promotion*, 14: 37–47.

O'Neill, C., Lamber, A., Linnell, R. and Warr-Wood, J. (1989) *Drama Guidelines*. London: Heinemann.

Parker, C. (1997) The relationship between speeding attitudes and speeding behaviour, in G. Grayson (ed.) *Behavioural Research in Road Safety VII*. Crowthorne: Transport Research Laboratory.

Parker, D., Manstead, A.S.R. and Stradling, S.G. (1995) Extending the theory of planned behaviour: the role of personal norm, *British Journal of Social Psychology*, 34: 127–37.

Parker, D., Manstead, A.S.R., Stradling, S.G., Reason, J.T. and Baxter, J.S. (1992) Intention to commit driving violations: an application of the theory of planned behaviour, *Journal of Applied Psychology*, 77: 94–101.

Petty, R.E. and Cacioppo, J.T. (1986) *Communication and Persuasion: Central and Peripheral Routes to Attitude Change*. New York: Springer.

Pless, I.B., Peckham, C.S. and Power, C. (1989) Predicting traffic injuries in childhood: a cohort analysis, *Journal of Pediatrics*, 115: 932–8.

Powney, J., Glissov, P. and Hall, S. (1995) *The Use of Theatre Tours in Road Safety Education: Drinking, Driving and Young People*, SCRE research report no. 66. Edinburgh: Scottish Council for Research in Education.

Quine, L., Rutter, D.R. and Arnold, L. (1998) Predicting and understanding safety helmet use among schoolboy cyclists: a comparison of the Theory of Planned Behaviour and the Health Belief Model, *Psychology and Health*, 13: 251–69.

Richard, R., van der Pligt, J. and de Vries, N. (1996) Anticipated affect and behavioral choice, *Basic and Applied Social Psychology*, 18: 111–29.

Roberts, I. (1993) Why have child pedestrian death rates fallen?, *British Medical Journal*, 306: 1737–9.

Russo, M.F., Stokes, G.S., Lahey, B.B. *et al.* (1993) A sensation seeking scale for children: further refinement and psychometric development, *Journal of Psychopathology and Behavioral Assessment*, 15: 69–86.

Rutter, D.R., Quine, L. and Chesham, D.J. (1995) Predicting safe riding behaviour and accidents: demography, beliefs, and behaviour in motorcycling safety, *Psychology and Health*, 10: 369–86.

Singh, A. and Spear, M. (1989) *Traffic Education: A Survey of Current Provision and Practice in Secondary Schools*, TRRL report no. CR115. Crowthorne: Transport and Road Research Laboratory.

Sissons Joshi, M., Beckett, K. and Macfarlane, A. (1994) Cycle helmet wearing in teenagers: do health beliefs influence behaviour?, *Archives of Disease in Childhood*, 71: 536–9.

Southwell, M.T., Carsten, O.M.J. and Tight, M.R. (1990) *Contributory Factors in Urban Road Accidents*. University of Leeds: Institute for Transport Studies.

Sparks, P. and Shepherd, R. (1992) Self-identity and the theory of planned behavior: assessing the role of identification with green consumerism, *Social Psychology Quarterly*, 55: 388–99.

Stasson, M. and Fishbein, M. (1990) The relationship between perceived risk and preventive action: a within-subjects analysis of perceived driving risk and intentions to wear seatbelts, *Journal of Applied Social Psychology*, 20: 1541–57.

Sutton, S. (1998) Predicting and explaining intentions and behavior: how well are we doing?, *Journal of Applied Social Psychology*, 28(15): 1317–38.

Telch, M.J., Miller, L.M., Killen, J.D., Cooke, S. and Maccoby, N. (1990) Long-term follow-up of a pilot project on smoking prevention with adolescents, *Journal of Behavioral Medicine*, 5: 1–8.

Thomson, J.A., Tolmie, A., Foot, H.C. and McLaren, B. (1996) *Child Development and the Aims of Road Safety Education*, Department of Transport Road Safety Research Report no. 1. London: Department of Transport.

Thuen, F. and Bendixen, M. (1996) The relationship between antisocial behaviour and injury-related behaviour among young Norwegian adolescents, *Health Education Research*, 9: 215–23.

Thuen, F. and Rise, J. (1994) Young adolescents' intention to use seatbelts: the role of attitudinal and normative beliefs, *Health Education Research*, 9(2): 215–23.

Tight, M.R. (1987) Accident involvement and exposure to risk for children as pedestrians on urban roads. PhD thesis, University of London.

Tight, M.R. (1996) A review of road safety research on children as pedestrians: how far can we go towards improving their safety?, *ATSS Research*, 20: 69–74.

Tight, M.R., Carsten, O.M.J., Kirby, H.R., Southwell, M.T. and Leake, G.R. (1990) Urban road traffic accidents: an in-depth study. Public Transport Research and Computing Eighteenth Summer Annual Meeting, Seminar G, University of Sussex, Brighton, September.

Triandis, H.C. (1977) *Interpersonal Behavior*. Monterey, CA: Brooks/Cole.

Wadsworth, M. (1987) Delinquency prediction and its uses: the experience of a 21 year follow-up study, *International Journal of Mental Health*, 7: 43–62.

Ward, H., Cave, B.L., Morrison, A., Allsop, R. and Evans, A. (1994) *Pedestrian Activity and Accident Risk*. Basingstoke: AA Foundation for Road Safety Research.

West, M.A. and Farr, J.L. (1989) Innovation at work: psychological perspectives, *Social Behaviour*, 4: 15–30.

West, R., Train, H., Junger, M., West, A. and Pickering, A. (1999) Accidents and problem behaviour, *The Psychologist*, 12: 395–7.

Whitebread, D. and Neilson, K. (1996) *Cognitive and Metacognitive Processes Underlying the Development of Children's Pedestrian Skills*, Department of Transport report no. S2/141 Child Development. London: HMSO.

Wittenbraker, J., Gibbs, B.L. and Kahle, L.R. (1983) Seat belt attitudes, habits and behaviours: an adaptive amendment to the Fishbein Model, *Journal of Applied Social Psychology*, 13(5): 406–21.

Zuckerman, M., Eysenck, S. and Eysenck, H.J. (1978) Sensation seeking in England and America: cross-cultural, age and sex comparisons, *Journal of Consulting and Clinical Psychology*, 46: 139–49.

10

LYN QUINE, DEREK RUTTER
AND LAURENCE ARNOLD

INCREASING CYCLE HELMET USE IN SCHOOL-AGE CYCLISTS: AN INTERVENTION BASED ON THE THEORY OF PLANNED BEHAVIOUR

This chapter presents an intervention to increase helmet use in school-age cyclists. The first section describes the statistics on pedal cycle accidents in young people and the evidence that helmets prevent or reduce head injury, and reviews other interventions to increase helmet use. The second section presents the theoretical framework we used to develop the intervention, the Theory of Planned Behaviour. The third section reports the development and evaluation of the intervention. The final section discusses the results and implications for further research.

1 Increasing helmet use in school-age cyclists

1.1 Pedal cycle casualties in young people and cycle helmet use

Pedal cycle accidents are a significant cause of accidental death and injury in children. In the UK in 1999 a total of 8403 school-age cyclists between 8 and 19 were killed or injured on the roads, representing almost 37 per cent of all injuries to cyclists (DETR 2000). In a recent paper (Quine *et al.* 1998) we reviewed casualties for child cyclists, showing that they are under-reported (Agran *et al.* 1990) and age-related (Jones 1989), and that boys are at higher risk than girls (Thomas *et al.* 1994; Towner *et al.* 1994). Cycling accidents to children occur most frequently on weekdays on journeys to and from school (Taylor 1989) and they often result in serious head and brain injuries (McDermott and Klug 1982; Wood and Milne 1988; Stutts *et al.* 1990). Few child cyclists wear helmets in countries where it is not legally mandatory (Cushman *et al.* 1990; Sissons Joshi *et al.* 1994). Cushman *et al.* (1990) report that only 2 per cent of 568 injured cyclists were wearing a helmet at the time of their injury although 13 per cent claimed to own one. Sissons-Joshi *et al.* (1994) found that only 13 per cent of their sample always wore a helmet and that rates of wearing decreased with increasing age. Other research seems to confirm this finding (DiGuiseppi *et al.* 1990; Stutts *et al.* 1990; Maimaris *et al.* 1994). Cycle helmets have been shown to prevent or reduce the effect of head injury (Dorsch *et al.* 1987; Thompson *et al.* 1989; McDermott *et al.* 1993; Maimaris *et al.* 1994; Pitt *et al.* 1994; Thomas *et al.* 1994; Thompson *et al.* 1996; Rivara *et al.* 2000; Thompson *et al.* 2000). In a recent editorial in the *British Medical Journal* based on a systematic review of five case control studies, Rivara *et al.* (2000) noted that helmets reduced the risk of head and brain injury by 63–88 per cent among cyclists of all ages. Four of the studies controlled for a number of important covariates. Helmets were equally effective in reducing injuries in accidents involving motor vehicles (69 per cent) and in accidents associated with falls and other causes (68 per cent). Injuries to the upper and mid-facial areas were also reduced (65 per cent).

1.2 Interventions to increase helmet use

A number of attempts have been made to increase helmet use among young cyclists using school-based interventions (Moore and Adair 1990; Pendergrast *et al.* 1992; Towner and Marvel 1992; Rouke 1994), local community programmes (Wood and Milne 1988; Bergman *et al.* 1990; Puczynski and Marshall 1992; Winn *et al.* 1992; Morris *et al.* 1994), physician advice (Cushman *et al.* 1991) and legislative and/or educational interventions (Cote *et al.* 1992; Dannenberg *et al.* 1993; Cameron *et al.* 1994). However, many of these campaigns have either failed outright or achieved only limited success (see Hillman 1993; Weiss 1994; Sibert 1996 for reviews). Weiss (1992), in a review of trends in children's bicycle helmet use, concluded that relatively modest school-based interventions appear to be the most effective. They do not have the problems associated with large-scale community-wide programmes, such as prohibitive running costs, reduced rates of bicycle use among young people, and difficulties with enforcement strategies (see Weiss 1992 for reviews; Hillman 1993).

In the UK no formal attempts have been made to promote helmet use among school-age cyclists and one must turn to countries such as the USA, Australia and New Zealand for examples. However, none of these has attempted to modify attitudes to helmet use using a theory-driven approach (see for example Moore and Adair 1990; Pendergrast *et al.* 1992). Instead they focus on helmet wearing as a 'common sense' practice and use strategies such as providing educational pamphlets, or giving audio/video presentations and lectures to increase awareness of helmets and the dangers of non-use.

There are other differences too between these studies and the one to be reported here: all involve elementary (junior) school children either exclusively or as a large part of their sample; none focuses exclusively on school-related cycling; and there is a reliance on helmet discount schemes, as if reducing the cost of buying a helmet will, in itself, increase helmet use. None the less a short review of these studies will provide a benchmark against which to judge the success of the present study.

Pendergrast and his colleagues (1992) conducted a year-long educational intervention in two elementary schools in Augusta, USA, in which they compared two types of intervention programme, one a traditional educational campaign and the other enhanced by meetings, 'bike clubs' and safety clinics. Although helmet *ownership* increased in both schools, only 9.3 per cent of the 'intensive' group actually wore a helmet after the programme, compared to a 6.8 per cent baseline user rate – an increase of just 2.5 per cent. A five-day intervention set in six elementary schools in Wisconsin, USA (Towner and Marvel 1992) was no more successful despite using 'fear appeal',[1] prizes and discount vouchers. The authors reported an increase in helmet *ownership* from 13 per cent to 27 per cent after a five-day programme, but no increase in observed helmet *use* (either immediately after the intervention or 19 weeks later). In contrast, a more elaborate intervention set in two intermediate schools in Auckland, New Zealand (Moore and Adair 1990) did achieve a degree of success. An initial (educational) intervention increased helmet use in the intervention school from 3.5 per cent to 14.4 per cent. The introduction of 'on the spot' prizes then increased it to 23.0 per cent, and final user rates 10 weeks after the intervention were reported to be 33.3 per cent. However, the authors acknowledged that the awarding of attractive prizes for 'good behaviour' was likely to be partly responsible for the second increase and that a serious bicycling accident involving a pupil at the intervention school was probably responsible for the final increase.

The effects of the accident on Moore and Adair's results can be gauged by comparison with a similar two-year long campaign conducted by Rouke (1994), which also featured a serious bicycling accident. Rouke's campaign was based in three elementary schools in Ontario, Canada, but also placed newspaper advertisements to publicize the programme and held public 'bicycle rodeos'. Local police carried out roadside spot checks (to reward helmet use) and it was possible to purchase subsidized helmets. Rouke notes that despite an initial 17-fold increase in helmet use provoked by the intervention (0.75 per cent to 12.80 per cent), more than 87 per cent of children still did not wear a helmet. Some time later, following a fatal bicycle accident involving a non-helmeted cyclist at the intervention school, helmet use rose dramatically to 51 per cent, though it quickly began to fall soon after. This suggests that a highly publicized bicycling accident is likely to have a noticeable but perhaps short-lived effect on helmet user rates.

A final study by Farley and her colleagues in Quebec (Farley *et al.* 1996) is described because it is the only one based, albeit loosely, on theory – in this case the PRECEDE framework and Rogers' diffusions of innovations theory (Green *et al.* 1980; Rogers 1983). These theories stress the importance of identifying factors likely to influence intentions to use helmets and the role of persuasive communication in bringing about change. In Farley *et al.*'s study, a 32 per cent increase in helmet use was observed by the end of four years. The intervention was three times more successful in the richer municipalities than in the poorer ones.

2 Theoretical perspective: the Theory of Planned Behaviour and the Elaboration Likelihood Model of Persuasion

2.1 The Theory of Planned Behaviour

In the following pages we report the development and evaluation of an intervention based on the TPB (Ajzen 1985, 1988, 1991) to promote the use of helmets among school-age cyclists. The TPB provides a theoretical account of the way in which attitude, subjective norm, perceived behavioural control and behavioural intention combine to predict behaviour and is described in the introduction to this volume. In an earlier book on its parent theory, the Theory of Reasoned Action, Fishbein and Ajzen (1975) discussed how such models might be used to change behaviour. They argued that successful behavioural change would occur only if the underlying attitudinal and normative beliefs that determine intentions were targeted. Within the TPB, beliefs about perceived behavioural control would also be included. Fishbein and Ajzen suggested three strategies to bring about belief change. The first involves creating new salient attitudinal and normative beliefs for a target population, the second making existing non-salient beliefs salient, and the third changing existing salient beliefs. However, beyond this the authors did not specify how to introduce new salient beliefs, to go about changing existing ones, or to choose the arguments to include in messages designed to modify particular salient beliefs (Eagly and Chaiken 1993: 200; Sutton, Chapter 11 in this volume). The Elaboration Likelihood Model of Persuasion (ELM: Petty and Cacioppo 1986a, 1986b) does provide some guidance on the processes involved in persuasion, and we therefore used it to provide insight into how to bring about change in beliefs that is enduring, resistant to counterpersuasion, and predictive of behaviour.

2.2 The Elaboration Likelihood Model of Persuasion

The Elaboration Likelihood Model of Persuasion (Petty and Cacioppo 1986b) describes a psychological process whereby cognitive responses to information bring about lasting attitude change, and defines the conditions under which this is likely to occur. The model proposes that there are two qualitatively different routes to persuasion: a 'central route' in which message recipients engage in cognitive elaboration of issue-relevant arguments contained in a persuasive message/advocacy, and a 'peripheral route' in which recipients are influenced by peripheral issues such as source credibility or attributional reasoning (Petty and Cacioppo 1986a, 1986b; Eagly and Chaiken 1993). By elaboration, Petty and Cacioppo mean the extent to which the individual is motivated to think carefully about the arguments contained in a persuasive communication. The authors identify *message-relevant thinking* as the mechanism that mediates central route processing. Thus if participants can be persuaded by the nature and quality of the message to engage in 'diligent consideration of issue-relevant arguments' (Petty *et al.* 1981), then elaboration likelihood is said to be high. This means that people are likely to attend to an appeal, attempt to access relevant information from both internal and external sources, scrutinize and make inferences about the message arguments in the light of other pertinent information, draw conclusions about the merits of the arguments based upon their own analyses, and derive an overall evaluation of, or attitude towards, them. Petty and Cacioppo believe that issue-relevant elaboration results in the new arguments being integrated into the individual's underlying belief structure. Thus 'central route' processing produces attitudes that have temporal persistence and are predictive of behaviour and resistant to change, while peripheral route processing is typified by absence of argument scrutiny and produces only temporary attitude change. The method represents an important alternative to traditional education-based persuasive attempts, which encourage participants to learn the contents of a message as if this will be sufficient in itself.

Petty and Cacioppo (1986b) argue that central route processing is more likely to occur when there is personal involvement with the central issues contained in a persuasive communication and when argument quality is high. Under these conditions, participants will generate a large number of favourable cognitive responses, which will increase the likelihood that the contents of the persuasive communication will produce lasting attitude change.

3 The intervention

The aim of the present study was to design and evaluate an intervention based on the TPB to strengthen the importance of behavioural and normative beliefs associated with helmet use and reduce the importance of perceptions of impediment, and thus promote helmet use among school-age cyclists. Development involved the five steps suggested by Sutton in Chapter 11: definition of target behaviour and population (Step 1); pilot study to elicit modal salient beliefs (Step 2); main study in which the components of the TPB are operationalized according to Ajzen and Fishbein's (1980) and Ajzen's (1991) recommendations in order to test the model (Step 3) and assess which beliefs best discriminate between helmet users and non-users (Step 4); and finally development and evaluation of an intervention to change the selected beliefs using a new sample (Step 5). The first four steps are described fully in an earlier paper (Quine *et al.* 1998).

3.1 Design and participants

The intervention design was a two by three mixed design: Condition (intervention/control) × Time (pre-intervention/immediately post-intervention/five-month follow-up). The participants were 97 adolescents aged between 11 and 15 years who regularly cycled to school but did not use a helmet. They were seen at school after agreeing to take part in a cycling survey. Participating schools were chosen at random from local authority lists, and nine out of twelve that agreed to take part were selected. The sole criterion was that the school should be situated in or near a large town or population centre to ensure that all participants experienced urban traffic conditions while travelling to school. The study involved three time points. At Time 1 information was obtained about participants' helmet use, intentions, normative, behavioural and control beliefs, helmet ownership, age and gender to ensure that only participants who did not currently use a helmet were included in the study. At Time 2 the intervention took place. Participants were randomly assigned to control or intervention conditions, and each was given a booklet containing the intervention materials. The booklets were designed to be as similar as possible in the format used for each message, the tasks involved, and the time required to respond to each one. After completing the tasks, each group filled in a questionnaire containing the normative, behavioural, control and intention items to evaluate the immediate effects of the intervention. At Time 3, five months later, a questionnaire based on the TPB was presented to participants, to evaluate the long-term effects of the intervention on beliefs, intention and behaviour. Participants were debriefed and the researcher agreed to provide each school with a report of the findings.

3.2 Materials

The materials for the intervention took the form of two five-page A5-size booklets.

Selecting the beliefs to be targeted

We selected the two behavioural, two normative and two control beliefs that had been shown by t-test to discriminate best between helmet users and non-users in our earlier research (Quine *et al.* 1998), and these beliefs provided the basis for the persuasive messages. The behavioural beliefs were 'Wearing a helmet while cycling to and from school would make me take care' and 'Wearing a helmet while cycling to and from school would protect my head in an accident.' The normative beliefs were 'My parents think that I should wear a helmet while cycling to and from school' and 'Most of the other cyclists at school think that I should wear a helmet while cycling to and from school.' The control beliefs were 'Even if I wanted to, I might not be able to wear a helmet while cycling to and from school because doing up and adjusting the straps is too much effort' and 'Even if I wanted to, I might not be able to wear a helmet while cycling to and from school because there is nowhere to keep it during lessons.'

Intervention condition booklets

The booklet given to the intervention group contained two paper and pencil tasks involving persuasive messages based on the six salient beliefs outlined above. The first task required participants to respond to and elaborate on persuasive messages contained in a series of flowcharts, and the second task consisted of a thought-listing procedure designed to encourage participants to recall and elaborate on the information provided in the messages. The messages took the form of question and answer flowcharts designed to ensure that the participants had to respond and give active consideration to the textual information (see Figure 10.1 for examples). There were five charts. The first two presented the positive behavioural outcomes associated with helmet use: 'taking care' and 'being protected in an accident'. The next two presented the perceived normative expectations of parents and other cyclists and were designed to make cyclists reconsider and elaborate on the reasons why parents would worry less if they wore a helmet and whether it was more important to protect their head or to worry about what other cyclists at school would think of them if they wore a helmet. The fifth chart presented two impediments to helmet use and was designed to encourage participants to consider ways of overcoming them.

Control condition booklets

The booklet for the control condition contained two paper and pencil tasks concerned with a hypothetical cycling proficiency and maintenance course and was designed to mimic the intervention booklet by presenting persuasive messages about behavioural and normative outcomes associated with attending such a course and solutions to practical difficulties that attendance might cause. Again the messages took the form of flowcharts (see Figure 10.2). The first two charts were concerned with behavioural outcomes by way of consideration of the advantages of attending the proposed course. The next two charts dealt with the normative expectations of two reference groups with respect to attendance: road safety experts and other cyclists.

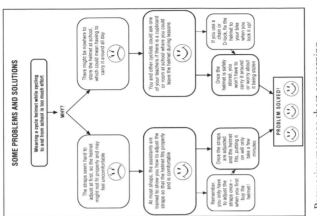

Persuasive message chart concerning beliefs about Perceived Behavioural Control 1 and 2, 'Impediments to helmet use'

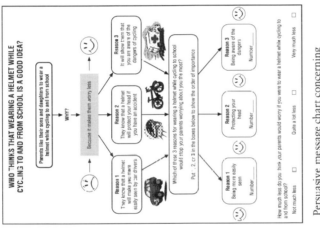
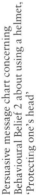
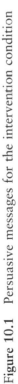

Persuasive message chart concerning Normative Belief 1 about using a helmet, 'Perceived parental expectations'

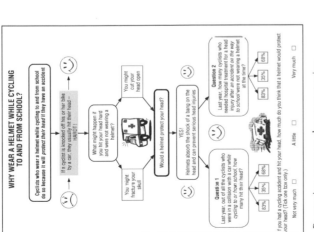

Persuasive message chart concerning Behavioural Belief 2 about using a helmet, 'Protecting one's head'

Figure 10.1 Persuasive messages for the intervention condition

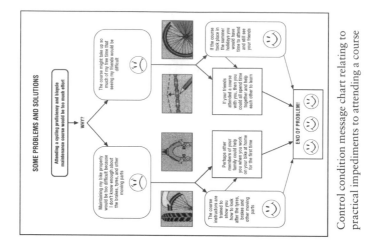

Control condition message chart relating to the normative expectations of other cyclists

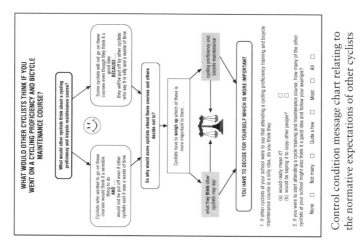

Control condition message chart relating to practical impediments to attending a course

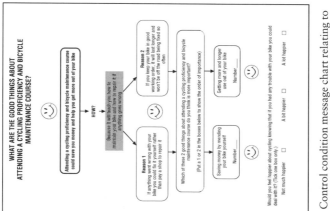

Control condition message chart relating to perceived behavioural outcomes

Figure 10.2 Persuasive messages for the control condition

The fifth chart was concerned with two practical impediments to attending a cycling proficiency training and bicycle maintenance course.

3.3 Measures

The measures used to evaluate the intervention were based on our previous research on predicting helmet use (Quine *et al.* 1998). Questionnaires based on the TPB were presented to the participants at Times 1, 2 and 3. At each time point, behavioural intention and the relevant behavioural, normative and control beliefs used to form the persuasive messages were measured and participants were asked whether they currently wore helmets. The two behavioural beliefs were computed from belief strength multiplied by outcome evaluation. Belief strength was assessed on seven-point unipolar scales from 1 'Extremely unlikely' to 7 'Extremely likely' and outcome evaluation was measured on bipolar scales from +3 'Extremely good' to −3 'Extremely bad' as Ajzen recommends (Ajzen 1991: 193). The two normative beliefs were computed from the normative statements multiplied by motivation to comply. Both were measured on seven-point scales from 1 'Extremely unlikely' to 7 'Extremely likely'. The control beliefs were measured on seven-point scales from 1 'Strongly disagree' to 7 'Strongly agree'. An overall perceived behavioural control item 'For me to wear a helmet when cycling to and from school would be (1) difficult . . . (7) easy' was also included. Intention was measured by a single item, 'I intend to wear a helmet while cycling to and from school in the future', scored from 1 'Extremely unlikely' to 7 'Extremely likely'. Helmet use was measured at Time 3 by a single dichotomous item 'Do you wear a helmet when cycling to and from school?' (Yes/No).

3.4 Statistical analyses

T-tests were used to examine whether there were any systematic differences between the intervention and control groups prior to the intervention. To evaluate the intervention itself, the effects of Group and Time on behavioural, normative, and control beliefs and intention were examined by analysis of covariance, adjusting for Time 1 scores: Group (Intervention/Control) by Time (Time 2/Time 3 with Time 1 covaried out). A chi-squared test examined the effects of the intervention on helmet use. Finally, differences between helmet users and non-users at Times 2 and 3 were analysed by two-way analysis of variance (users/non-users by Time 2/Time 3).

3.5 Results

Time 1 (initial assessment)
A total of 189 boys and 51 girls took part in the preliminary assessment. Differences in the number of males and females reflected the proportions of

each sex who cycled to school. One school withdrew its 55 pupils from the study, and staff at four other schools asked that cyclists over the age of 14 (33 boys and 7 girls) be excluded from further involvement because of examination pressure. Of the original 240 cyclists, this left 118 boys and 27 girls. A further 33 cyclists were then excluded from future involvement after declaring themselves to be helmet users. After these adjustments 112 cyclists were available to take part in the intervention and arrangements were made to involve them at Time 2.

Time 2 (immediately post-intervention)
Of the participants at Time 1, 8 were absent at Time 2, leaving 104. Each participant was randomly assigned to either the intervention condition or the control condition. Data from 7 of the 104 was discarded: 3 had rendered one or both of their questionnaires unusable and 4 were now helmet users, leaving data from 97 participants (75 boys and 22 girls) to be collated, 48 in the intervention condition and 49 in the control condition. The sample at this stage ranged in age from 11 to 14 years, with a mean of 12.3: 18 of the participants were aged 11, 70 were aged 12 or 13, and 9 were aged 14. The sexes were equally represented in all age groups; 51 of the participants (52.6 per cent) owned a helmet, proportionately more girls (63.6 per cent) than boys (49.3 per cent).

Time 3 (five-month follow-up)
Five months later, at Time 3, all participants completed a further questionnaire. At this time, 50 cyclists said they owned a helmet (51.5 per cent of the sample), 30 in the intervention group and 20 in the control group. Although helmet ownership among boys remained constant at 49.3 per cent across the sessions, it fell slightly among girls, with 1 fewer at Time 2 claiming to own a helmet; 13 (59.1 per cent) still owned a helmet at Time 3.

*Effects of the intervention on behavioural, normative
and control beliefs*
Before the main analyses were carried out, composite variables were constructed from the constituent items. Each belief strength item was multiplied by its corresponding outcome evaluation to create a product, and the two normative belief items were computed by multiplying each of the normative statements by its corresponding motivation to comply. The two control beliefs and the overall perceived behavioural control items were single item statements. The first analysis examined whether there were any systematic differences in normative, behavioural or control beliefs or behavioural intention between groups prior to the intervention at Time 1. This was done by t-test. No significant differences were found. The second analysis examined the effects of the intervention on beliefs and intention as described in the Design and Method section. The means are given in Table 10.1, together

Table 10.1 Effects of group and time: analysis of covariance

	Means								F ratios		
	Time 2				Time 3						
	Intervention		Control		Intervention		Control		Group	Time	Interaction
	Mean	SD	Mean	SD	Mean	SD	Mean	SD			
Behavioural Belief 1 My wearing a helmet while cycling to and from school would make me take care	10.9	9.0	5.1	6.8	8.5	6.6	4.9	8.0	10.5**	0.7	2.3
Behavioural Belief 2 My wearing a helmet while cycling to and from school would protect my head if I had an accident	11.6	10.4	11.2	11.8	12.9	9.3	10.4	11.0	0.3	1.9	1.1
Normative Belief 1 My parents think that I should wear a helmet while cycling to and from school	29.2	13.0	18.2	14.6	24.9	13.0	17.0	13.0	16.5***	0.9	1.1
Normative Belief 2 Most of the other cyclists at my school think that I should wear a helmet while cycling to and from school	14.7	15.4	8.9	9.8	12.0	10.4	8.6	8.2	4.9*	0.4	0.9
Control Belief 1 Even if I wanted to, I might not be able to wear a helmet while cycling to and from school because adjusting and/or doing up the straps is too much effort	4.6	1.8	3.9	1.8	4.8	1.7	4.3	1.9	3.4	0.8	0.1
Control Belief 2 Even if I wanted to, I might not be able to wear a helmet while cycling to and from school because there is nowhere to keep it during lessons	3.9	2.0	3.6	2.1	3.9	1.9	3.5	2.3	1.2	0.0	0.1
Perceived Behavioural Control For me to wear a helmet while cycling to and from school would be . . . (difficult – easy)	4.8	1.8	3.8	2.1	4.4	2.0	3.7	2.0	6.4*	0.1	0.8
Intention I intend to wear a helmet while cycling to and from school in the future	3.5	2.2	2.4	1.6	3.8	2.0	2.9	2.1	5.7*	0.3	0.5

Notes: * p < 0.05   ** p < 0.01   *** p < 0.001

with the F ratios for Group, Time, and Group by Time interactions. For five of the eight measures, there were significant main effects for Group, but there were none for Time and there were no Group by Time interactions. For all the significant main effects of Group, the intervention group had higher scores than the control group, on both occasions. The non-significant trend for the three remaining measures was the same.

Effects of the intervention on helmet use
The third analysis tested the hypothesis that the persuasive advocacy would lead to an increase in helmet use in the intervention group. A chi-squared test was conducted to examine the association between helmet use at Time 3 and group, and it revealed a significant effect. The results are shown in Table 10.2. Of the 48 participants in the intervention group 12 (25 per cent) now used a helmet, while none of the control group did so. This suggests that the persuasive advocacy presented to the intervention group was effective in increasing helmet use.

Table 10.2　Helmet use at Time 3 follow-up by group

Group	Uses a helmet at Time 3		Does not use a helmet at Time 3	
	%	n	%	n
Intervention (n = 48)	25	12	75	36
Control (n = 49)	0	0	100	49

Notes: Chi-squared = 11.8 df 1 $p < 0.001$

Differences between helmet users and non-users at Time 2 and 3
The final analysis addressed the question of whether changes in behaviour among the intervention group could be explained by changes in beliefs. To test whether helmet users in the intervention group differed from non-users in their beliefs and intention after the intervention, and whether the differences, if any, were stable over time, the data were analysed by two-way analysis of variance: users/non-users by Time 2/Time 3. The means are given in Table 10.3, together with the F ratios. Users differed significantly from non-users for five of the measures; for two of the five there were significant main effects of time; but there were no significant interactions. Whenever users differed from non-users, the users' scores were higher on both occasions; and whenever there was a significant effect of time, the Time 3 scores were lower than the Time 2 scores.

	Means								F ratios		
	Time 2				Time 3						
	Helmet users (n = 12)		Non-users (n = 36)		Helmet users (n = 12)		Non-users (n = 36)		Group	Time	Interaction
	Mean	SD	Mean	SD	Mean	SD	Mean	SD			
Behavioural Belief 1 My wearing a helmet while cycling to and from school would make me take care	15.8	6.6	9.3	9.2	10.7	5.8	7.7	6.7	4.4*	8.0**	2.2
Behavioural Belief 2 My wearing a helmet while cycling to and from school would protect my head if I had an accident	15.6	7.3	10.3	11.0	14.5	7.4	12.3	9.9	2.1	0.1	0.7
Normative Belief 1 My parents think that I should wear a helmet while cycling to and from school	39.3	10.3	25.9	12.2	36.4	10.4	21.0	11.5	22.8***	2.7	0.2
Normative Belief 2 Most of the other cyclists at my school think that I should wear a helmet while cycling to and from school	24.2	16.1	11.6	14.0	16.3	14.5	10.6	8.4	6.4*	4.5*	2.7
Control Belief 1 Even if I wanted to, I might not be able to wear a helmet while cycling to and from school because adjusting and/or doing up the straps is too much effort	5.2	1.9	4.4	1.8	5.1	1.7	4.7	1.7	1.3	0.2	0.6
Control Belief 2 Even if I wanted to, I might not be able to wear a helmet while cycling to and from school because there is nowhere to keep it during lessons	3.9	2.4	3.9	1.8	3.5	2.0	4.0	1.8	0.2	0.3	0.5
Perceived Behavioural Control For me to wear a helmet while cycling to and from school would be . . . (difficult – easy)	5.6	1.6	4.6	1.8	5.3	1.8	4.0	1.9	5.0*	1.4	0.2
Intention I intend to wear a helmet while cycling to and from school in the future	5.3	2.0	2.9	1.9	5.7	1.6	3.2	1.7	24.2***	1.0	0.0

Notes: $* p < 0.05$ $** p < 0.01$ $*** p < 0.001$

4 Discussion: implications for theory, policy and practice

The study set out to design and evaluate a longitudinal intervention, based on the TPB (Ajzen 1985, 1988, 1991), to promote the use of protective helmets by school-age cyclists. Beliefs identified in our previous empirical work using the TPB (Ajzen 1985) and shown to predict intention and helmet use were selected to inform a series of persuasive messages intended to influence the beliefs of young cyclists who did not use helmets. The results show that the intervention was successful in promoting a positive evaluation of the behavioural and normative outcomes of helmet use among message recipients compared to control participants, and, to a lesser extent, in decreasing the salience of factors affecting perceptions of behavioural control. After covarying out scores at Time 1, the intervention group were significantly more positive than the control group on four of the seven belief measures and in their intentions to use a helmet. These differences were evident five months after the intervention, indicating lasting attitude change. There was a significant increase in reported helmet use in the intervention group, but not in the control group: 12 intervention participants (25 per cent) now wore a helmet, but none of the 49 control participants. Two-way analysis of variance showed that in the intervention group helmet users differed significantly from non-users for five of the eight measures, suggesting that changes in behaviour were supported by changes in beliefs.

4.1 Behavioural beliefs

Intervention participants were more likely than control participants to endorse the belief that wearing a helmet would make them take care. However, there was no significant difference between groups in the belief that helmet use would protect cyclists' heads if they had an accident, though there was a trend in the expected direction, with message recipients endorsing the belief marginally more after the intervention and again five months later. That this belief did not also show a significant change was disappointing, though one should not underestimate the size of the task confronting one short intervention. Changing attitudes and health behaviours is notoriously difficult, and changing young people's perceptions of a health risk they probably believe they are less likely to experience than others is likely to be particularly difficult (Weinstein 1980).

4.2 Normative beliefs

Beliefs about parental expectation were one of the most powerful discriminators between the intervention and control groups, showing perhaps that perceptions of what significant others think we should do may be of more importance than our own beliefs when performing preventive health behaviours in public or where it is perceived that the consequences of failing to carry out the behaviour may affect the lives of referent others. Though reviews of the TPB have found that the normative component generally has the weakest links to intention and behaviour (Godin and Kok 1996; Armitage and Conner in press), a number of other studies attempting to explain health-related decisions have found subjective norm to be more important than attitude (Lacy 1981; Boyd and Wandersman 1991; Rutter 2000). Parker *et al.* (1996), in an intervention study that attempted to modify drivers' beliefs and attitudes to exceeding the speed limit using experimental videos, also found evidence in favour of the subjective norm. Videos using the concept of normative beliefs, and focusing on the disapproval of important others for speeding, were more successful in bringing about changes in general attitudes towards speeding than videos focusing on behavioural beliefs or control beliefs. The pattern of results also reflects findings from two other studies of cycling. Both Pendergrast *et al.* (1992) and Hu *et al.* (1993) found parents to be a powerful influence on young cyclists' helmet use.

4.3 Control beliefs and perceived behavioural control

Despite a trend in the predicted direction, the groups did not differ significantly in their endorsement of either of the two control beliefs. Message recipients were less likely than control participants to perceive difficulties in adjusting or doing up the straps as an impediment to helmet use, but the differences did not quite reach significance (p = 0.06). The intervention also failed to reduce intervention participants' perception of the problems of carrying a helmet round during lessons, although again there was a trend in the predicted direction. The failure to persuade participants fully that they can overcome these problems may derive from the fact that they are genuine impediments (see DiGuiseppi *et al.* 1990; Otis *et al.* 1992; Sissons Joshi *et al.* 1994) and ones that are hard to overcome.

The perception that using a helmet while cycling to school would be easy *was*, however, endorsed significantly more by message recipients than control participants across times of assessment. Because this belief was not specifically targeted by the persuasive advocacy it can be viewed as an overall evaluation of the impediments to helmet use. It has been argued by Ajzen (Ajzen and Madden 1986; Ajzen 1988) that these impediments constitute belief-based measures of control, which inform *overall* perceptions of behavioural control. The findings reported here support this contention, providing further support for the TPB.

4.4 Behavioural intentions

In the same way that the efficacy of the persuasive messages concerning impediments to helmet use were reflected in the increased perceptions of behavioural control among message recipients, so the increase in behavioural intentions provides an evaluation of the persuasive advocacy. Intention was not targeted in the intervention, yet message recipients expressed a stronger intention to engage in helmet use than did control participants. This is consistent with Ajzen's (1988) claim that beliefs about behavioural and normative outcomes and perceptions of control are the determinants of intention.

4.5 The effects of the intervention on behaviour

The intervention succeeded in persuading 12 of the 48 message recipients to wear a helmet regularly when cycling to school. The beliefs of the participants whose behaviour changed were also shown to differ significantly in levels of belief endorsement. This rate of success compares favourably with other promotional campaigns, many of which have used repeated intervention sessions or continuing programmes to promote helmet use (see for example Pendergrast *et al.* 1992; Towner and Marvel 1992; Rouke 1994). Even a four-year campaign in Quebec reported by Farley *et al.* (1996) achieved only a 32 per cent increase in helmet use. Moreover, helmet use among the participants in the study reported here was measured five months after the intervention, indicating that it was sustained over time. We believe this success occurred because the intervention set out to change beliefs and behaviour using a *theory-based* approach, rather than the more traditional education and advisory approaches that campaigns have normally used. Runyan and Runyan (1991), examining the issue of helmet promotion among young cyclists, point out that behaviour change is rarely effected solely by providing education and information, and this is borne out by the failure of many promotional campaigns. Winn *et al.* (1992), for example, using an educational and advisory approach, produced only a short-lived change in behaviour among young cyclists, user rates falling back to zero shortly after the end of the programme. The results of our study show that enduring changes in health behaviours such as using a safety helmet can be brought about by targeting salient health beliefs. Like many other findings reported in this volume, our results thus confirm that social cognition models such as the TPB have an important role to play in the design of interventions to promote healthy behaviours.

Note

1 Eggs, with or without a protective (egg carton) helmet and representing the human skull, were dropped to demonstrate the protection afforded by helmets and the effect of an impact.

References

Agran, P.F., Castillo, D.N. and Winn, D.G. (1990) Limitations of data compiled from police accident reports on pediatric pedestrian and bicycle motor vehicle events, *Accident Analysis and Prevention*, 22(4): 361–70.

Ajzen, I. (1985) From intentions to actions: a theory of planned behaviour, in J. Kuhl and J. Beckman (eds) *Action Control: From Cognition to Behaviour*. Heidelberg: Springer.

Ajzen, I. (1988) *Attitudes, Personality and Behavior*. Milton Keynes: Open University Press.

Ajzen, I. (1991) The Theory of Planned Behavior, *Organizational Behavior and Human Decision Processes*, 50: 179–211.

Ajzen, I. and Fishbein, M. (eds) (1980) *Understanding Attitudes and Predicting Social Behavior*. Englewood Cliffs, NJ: Prentice-Hall.

Ajzen, I. and Madden, T.J. (1986) Prediction of goal-directed behavior: attitudes, intention, and perceived behavioral control, *Journal of Experimental Social Psychology*, 22: 453–74.

Armitage, C.J. and Conner, M. (in press) Efficacy of the theory of planned behaviour: a meta-analytic review, *British Journal of Social Psychology*.

Bergman, A.B., Rivara, F.P., Richards, D.D. and Rogers, L.W. (1990) The Seattle Children's bicycle helmet campaign, *American Journal of Diseases of Children*, 144(6): 727–31.

Boyd, B. and Wandersman, A. (1991) Predicting undergraduate condom use with the Fishbein and Ajzen and the Triandis Attitude-Behaviour models: implications for public health interventions, *Journal of Applied Social Psychology*, 21(22): 1810–30.

Cameron, M.H., Vulcan, A.P., Finch, C.F. and Newstead, S.V. (1994) Mandatory bicycle helmet use following a decade of helmet promotion in Victoria, Australia – an evaluation, *Accident Analysis and Prevention*, 26: 325–37.

Cote, T.R., Sacks, J.J., Lambert-Huber, D.A. *et al.* (1992) Bicycle helmet use among Maryland children: effect of legislation and education, *Pediatrics*, 89(6): 1216–20.

Cushman, R., Down, J., MacMillan, N. and Waclawik, H. (1990) Bicycle-related injuries: a survey in a paediatric emergency department, *Canadian Medical Association Journal*, 143: 108–12.

Cushman, R., Down, J., MacMillan, N. and Waclawik, H. (1991) Helmet promotion in the emergency room following a bicycle injury: a randomised trial, *Pediatrics*, 88: 43–7.

Dannenberg, A.L., Gielen, A.C., Beilensen, P.L., Wilson, M.H. and Joffe, A. (1993) Bicycle helmet laws and educational campaigns: an evaluation of strategies to increase children's helmet use, *American Journal of Public Health*, 83(5): 667–74.

Department of the Environment, Transport and the Regions (DETR) (2000) *Road Accidents Great Britain 1999*. London: The Stationery Office.

DiGuiseppi, C.G., Rivara, F.P. and Koepsall, T.D. (1990) Attitudes toward bicycle helmet ownership and use by school-age children, *American Journal of Diseases of Children*, 144: 83–6.

Dorsch, M., Woodward, A.J. and Somers, R.L. (1987) Do bicycle safety helmets reduce the severity of head injuries in real crashes?, *Accident Analysis and Prevention*, 20: 447–58.

Eagly, A.H. and Chaiken, S. (1993) *The Psychology of Attitudes*. New York: Harcourt Brace and Jovanovich.

Farley, C., Haddad, S. and Brown, B. (1996) The effect of a four-year program promoting bicycle helmet use among children in Quebec, *American Journal of Public Health*, 86(1): 46–51.

Fishbein, M. and Ajzen, I. (1975) *Belief, Attitude, Intention and Behavior: An Introduction to Theory and Research*. Reading, MA: Addison-Wesley.

Godin, G. and Kok, G. (1996) The Theory of Planned Behavior: a review of its applications to health-related behaviors, *American Journal of Health Promotion*, 11(2): 87–98.

Green, L.W., Kreuter, M., Deed, S. and Partridge, K. (1980) *Health Education Planning: A Diagnostic Approach*. Palo Alto, CA: Mayfield.

Hillman, M. (1993) *Cycle Helmets: The Case For and Against*. Policy Studies Institute Report. Dorset: Blackmore Press.

Hu, X., Wesson, D.E., Parkin, P.C., Chipman, M.L. and Spence, L.J. (1993) Parental attitudes toward legislation for helmet use by child cyclists, *Canadian Journal of Public Health*, 85(2): 121–4.

Jones, D. (1989) Child casualties in road accidents, in Department of Transport (ed.) *Road Accidents Great Britain 1989: The Casualty Report*. London: HMSO.

Lacy, W.B. (1981) The influence of attitudes and current friends on drug use intentions, *Journal of Social Psychology*, 113: 65–76.

McDermott, F.T. and Klug, G.L. (1982) Differences in head injuries of pedal cyclist and motorcyclist casualties in Victoria, *Medical Journal of Australia*, 2: 30–2.

McDermott, F.T., Lane, J.C., Brazenon, G.A. and Debney, E.A. (1993) The effectiveness of bicycle helmets: a study of 1710 casualties, *Journal of Trauma*, 34: 835–45.

Maimaris, C., Summers, C.L., Browning, C. and Palmer, C.R. (1994) Injury patterns in cyclists attending an accident and emergency department: a comparison of helmet wearers and non-wearers, *British Medical Journal*, 308: 1537–40.

Moore, D.W. and Adair, V. (1990) Effects of a school-based education programme on safety helmet usage by 11- to 13-year old cyclists, *Educational Psychology*, 10(1): 73–8.

Morris, B.A., Trimble, N.E. and Fendley, S.J. (1994) Increasing bicycle helmet use in the community: measuring response to a wide-scale effort, *Canadian Family Physician*, 40: 1126–31.

Otis, J., Lesage, D., Godin, G. *et al.* (1992) Predicting and reinforcing children's intentions to wear protective helmets while bicycling, *Public Health Reports – Hyatsville*, 107: 283–7.

Parker, D., Stradling, S.G. and Manstead, A.S.R. (1996) Modifying beliefs and attitudes to exceeding the speed limit: an intervention study based on the theory of planned behavior, *Journal of Applied Social Psychology*, 26(1): 1–19.

Pendergrast, R.A., Ashworth, C.S., DuRant, R.H. and Litaker, M. (1992) Correlates of children's bicycle helmet use and short term failure of school-level interventions, *Pediatrics*, 90(3): 354–8.

Petty, R.E. and Cacioppo, J.T. (1986a) *Communication and Persuasion: Central and Peripheral Routes to Attitude Change*. New York: Springer.

Petty, R.E. and Cacioppo, J.T. (1986b) The elaboration likelihood model of persuasion, in L. Berkowitz (ed.) *Advances in Experimental Psychology*, 19. London: Academic Press.

Petty, R.E., Cacioppo, J.T. and Goldman, R. (1981) Personal involvement as a determinant of argument-based persuasion, *Journal of Personality and Social Psychology*, 41(5): 847–55.

Pitt, W.R., Thomas, S., Nixon, J. *et al.* (1994) Trends in head injuries among child bicyclists, *British Medical Journal*, 308: 177–8.

Puczynski, M. and Marshall, D.A. (1992) Helmets! All the pros wear them, *American Journal of Diseases of Children*, 146: 1465–7.

Quine, L., Rutter, D.R. and Arnold, L. (1998) Predicting and understanding safety helmet use among schoolboy cyclists: a comparison of the Theory of Planned Behaviour and the Health Belief Model, *Psychology and Health*, 13: 251–69.

Rivara, F.P., Thompson, D.C. and Thompson, R.S. (2000) Bicycle helmets: it's time to use them, *British Medical Journal*, 321: 1035–6.

Rogers, E.M. (1983) *Diffusion of Innovations*, 3rd edn. New York: Free Press.

Rouke, L.L. (1994) Bicycle helmet use among schoolchildren: impact of a community education programme and a cycling fatality, *Canadian Family Physician*, 40: 1116–24.

Runyan, C.W. and Runyan, D.K. (1991) How can physicians get kids to wear bicycle helmets? A prototypic challenge in injury prevention, *American Journal of Public Health*, 81(8): 972–3.

Rutter, D.R. (2000) Attendance and reattendance for breast cancer screening: a prospective three year test of the Theory of Planned Behaviour, *British Journal of Health Psychology*, 5: 1–13.

Sibert, J.R. (1996) Children and cycle helmets: the case for, *Child: Care, Health and Development*, 22(2): 99–103.

Sissons Joshi, M., Beckett, K. and Macfarlane, A. (1994) Cycle helmet wearing in teenagers: do health beliefs influence behaviour?, *Archives of Disease in Childhood*, 71: 536–9.

Stutts, J.C., Williamson, J.E., Whitley, T. and Sheldon, F.C. (1990) Bicycle accidents and injuries: a pilot study comparing hospital- and police-reported data, *Accident Analysis and Prevention*, 22: 67–78.

Taylor, S. (1989) Pedal cycle casualties, in Department of Transport (ed.) *Road Accidents Great Britain 1989: The Casualty Report*. London: HMSO.

Thomas, S., Acton, C., Nixon, J. *et al.* (1994) Effectiveness of bicycle helmets in preventing head injury in children: case-control study, *British Medical Journal*, 308: 173–6.

Thompson, D.C., Rivara, F.P. and Thompson, R. (2000) Helmets for preventing head and facial injuries in bicyclists (Cochrane Review), in *The Cochrane Library*, 4. Oxford: Update Software.

Thompson, D.C., Rivara, F.P. and Thompson, R.S. (1996) Effectiveness of bicycle safety helmets in preventing head injuries: a case-control study, *Journal of the American Medical Association*, 276: 1968–73.

Thompson, R.S., Rivara, F.P. and Thompson, D.C. (1989) A case-control study on the effectiveness of bicycle safety helmets, *New England Journal of Medicine*, 320: 1361–7.

Towner, E.M., Jarvis, S.N., Walsh, S.S. and Aynsley-Green, A. (1994) Measuring exposure to injury risk in schoolchildren aged 11–14, *British Medical Journal*, 308: 449–52.

Towner, P. and Marvel, M.K. (1992) A school-based intervention to increase the use of bicycle helmets, *Family Medicine*, 24(2): 156–8.

Weinstein, N.D. (1980) Unrealistic optimism about future life events, *Journal of Personality and Social Psychology*, 39(5): 806–20.

Weiss, B.D. (1992) Trends in bicycle helmet use by children: 1985 to 1990, *Pediatrics*, 89(1): 78–80.

Weiss, B.D. (1994) Bicycle-related head injuries, *Clinics in Sports Medicine*, 13(1): 99–112.

Winn, G.L., Jones, D.F. and Bonk, C.J. (1992) Taking it to the streets: helmet use and bicycle safety as components of inner-city youth development, *Clinical Pediatrics*, 31(11): 672–7.

Wood, T. and Milne, P. (1988) Head injuries to pedal cyclists and the promotion of helmet use in Victoria, Australia, *Accident Analysis and Prevention*, 20(3): 177–85.

11

STEPHEN SUTTON

USING SOCIAL COGNITION MODELS TO DEVELOP HEALTH BEHAVIOUR INTERVENTIONS: PROBLEMS AND ASSUMPTIONS

Social cognition models are widely used to study health behaviours (Conner and Norman 1996). Among the most popular are the Theory of Reasoned Action (Fishbein and Ajzen 1975; Ajzen and Fishbein 1980) and its extension, the Theory of Planned Behaviour (Ajzen 1991). Increasingly, they are being used as the basis for health behaviour interventions, as this volume and other authors have demonstrated (for example, Hardeman et al. submitted). However, although these theories appear to have direct implications for the development of such interventions, translation of theoretical postulates and empirical findings derived mainly from non-experimental studies of the theories into effective interventions is far from straightforward. This final chapter provides a detailed examination of problems that arise and assumptions that are implicit in this translation process. Wherever possible, when problems are identified, recommendations are made for research and practice. Although the discussion focuses on the TRA and the TPB, which have special problems of their own, some of the comments are also applicable to other models of health behaviour.

1 The Theory of Reasoned Action

According to the TRA, intention is the immediate determinant of behaviour. Intention, in turn, is determined by attitude towards the behaviour and subjective norm; the relative contribution of these two components may differ for different behaviours and different populations. Attitude towards the behaviour is determined by the *salient behavioural beliefs* (behavioural beliefs relating to salient outcomes of the behaviour). Behavioural beliefs have two components: belief strength (*b*) and outcome evaluation (*e*). These are assumed to combine multiplicatively. We use the notation *be* to denote belief strength multiplied by outcome evaluation for a single behavioural belief. The sum of the *be*'s for the salient behavioural beliefs (which we refer to as *indirect attitude*) is assumed to determine attitude towards the behaviour (*direct attitude*). Subjective norm is determined by the *salient normative beliefs* (normative beliefs concerning salient referents). Like behavioural beliefs, normative beliefs have two components: belief strength (*n*) and motivation to comply (*m*), which are assumed to combine multiplicatively. Let *nm* denote belief strength multiplied by motivation to comply for a single normative belief. The sum of the *nm*'s for the salient normative beliefs (*indirect subjective norm*) is assumed to determine subjective norm (*direct subjective norm*). For present purposes, we assume that the behaviour in question is a recommended health-related action (for example use a condom consistently with new sexual partners) and that the aim of an intervention is to increase intention and therefore behaviour.

According to the TRA, there are three strategies for achieving this aim:

1 Change existing salient beliefs.
2 Make existing non-salient beliefs salient.
3 Create new salient beliefs.

It is assumed that there is a limit on the number of beliefs that are salient at any one time (Fishbein and Ajzen 1975: 218–22). Implementation of the second and third strategies may therefore have the consequence of making existing salient beliefs non-salient. In all three cases, the net effect of any changes or additions must be to increase indirect attitude or indirect subjective norm, otherwise the desired increases in intention and behaviour would not be expected to ensue.

This chapter follows previous discussions of using the TRA to develop interventions (for example Fishbein and Middlestadt 1989) by focusing on the first of the three strategies.[1] Note that beliefs can be modified by changing either or both of their two components. Table 11.1 lists the possible ways of changing behavioural and normative beliefs and gives examples for condom use.

2 Steps in developing a TRA-based intervention

Using the TRA to develop a health behaviour intervention involves the following sequence of steps. A similar approach will be necessary with other social cognition models.

Table 11.1   Ways of changing existing beliefs

(a) Increase belief strength for beliefs about positive outcomes
(for example increase belief strength for the belief that using a condom will reduce the risk of becoming infected with HIV)

(b) Increase the evaluation of positive outcomes that are perceived to be likely
(for example increase the evaluation of the outcome 'having a reduced risk of becoming infected with HIV', assuming that this outcome is perceived to be likely)

(c) Decrease the evaluation of positive outcomes that are perceived to be unlikely
(for example if the outcome 'increases my sexual stamina' is seen as salient and positive but unlikely, then decrease the evaluation of this outcome, that is, convince recipients that an increase in sexual stamina is not as desirable as they thought)

(d) Decrease belief strength for beliefs about negative outcomes
(for example decrease belief strength for the belief that using a condom will spoil one's sexual pleasure)

(e) Increase (that is, make more positive) the evaluation of negative outcomes that are perceived to be likely
(for example if a reduction in sexual pleasure is seen as a likely consequence of using a condom, then increase the evaluation of this outcome, that is, persuade recipients that a reduction in sexual pleasure is not as undesirable as they thought)

(f) Decrease (that is, make more negative) the evaluation of negative outcomes that are perceived to be unlikely
(for example if the outcome 'causes a skin rash' is seen as a salient but unlikely consequence of using a condom, then decrease this evaluation, that is, persuade recipients that having a skin rash in that part of the body is not just bad but very bad)

(g) Increase belief strength for normative beliefs
(for example increase belief strength for recipients' belief that their sexual partner – or other significant referents – would want them to use a condom)

(h) Increase motivation to comply with referents who approve of the behaviour
(for example if current sexual partner is identified as a salient referent who approves of condom use, persuade recipients that they want to do what their current sexual partner wants them to do)

(i) Decrease motivation to comply with referents who disapprove of the behaviour
(for example if parents are identified as salient referents who disapprove of condom use, persuade recipients that they do not want to do what their parents want them to do)

Note: (a)–(f) refer to behavioural beliefs and (g)–(i) to normative beliefs. These strategies assume the use, and validity, of Fishbein and Ajzen's recommended scoring scheme: symmetric bipolar scales with a midpoint of zero for belief strength and outcome evaluation, unipolar scales for motivation to comply. Fishbein and Ajzen (1975: 401) also state that subjective norm can be targeted *directly*, but this seems inconsistent with the assumption that subjective norm is determined by normative beliefs.

Step 1

The first step is to define the target behaviour and the target population. The relative importance of attitude and subjective norm in determining intention and the salient beliefs that underlie these components may differ for different behaviours (for example using condoms with a new sexual partner versus using condoms with a regular partner) and different populations (for example heterosexual men or gay men).

Step 2

The second step is to conduct an elicitation study to identify the *modal salient beliefs* with respect to the target behaviour in a sample of people drawn from the target population. Those beliefs that are elicited first in response to open-ended questions such as 'What do you see as the advantages of your using condoms with new sexual partners?' are assumed to be salient for the individual. Those elicited most frequently in the sample are designated the modal salient beliefs.

Step 3

The next step is to conduct a study in a second sample from the target population in which all the TRA variables, including the modal salient beliefs, are assessed using closed-ended questions worded according to Ajzen and Fishbein's (1980) recommendations. We shall refer to this second study as the *main study*. In the analysis, intention is regressed on attitude and subjective norm in order to estimate the relative contribution of these two determinants. The findings are used to decide whether the proposed intervention should target the attitudinal component only, the normative component only, or both components. The other links specified by the model may also be tested.

Step 4

The next step is to use the same data set to identify the beliefs that best discriminate between intenders and non-intenders (or between those who subsequently perform the behaviour and those who do not). This is usually done by dividing the sample into two groups and comparing them on each of the relevant measures in turn, for example by conducting a series of t-tests.

Step 5

The final step is to develop an intervention designed to change these key beliefs, and to evaluate this intervention using the TRA measures in a third sample drawn from the target population.

3 The Theory of Planned Behaviour

The same sequence can be used to develop an intervention based on the TPB, but several complications arise in this case. Additional questions need to be included in the pilot study to elicit salient control beliefs and in the main study to measure the modally salient control beliefs and perceived behavioural control (PBC). The regression analysis in the main study will include PBC as a predictor as well as attitude and subjective norm. Unlike the TRA, the TPB does not assume that intention is the sole proximal determinant of behaviour. It is quite consistent with the TPB for intention to turn out to be only a weak predictor of subsequent behaviour. If this proves to be the case, and if PBC is a relatively strong predictor, the researcher may decide that the intervention should target PBC and its putative determinants. However, this conclusion is problematic because of the causal ambiguity of the independent predictive effect of PBC on behaviour. Consider the following quotation from Ajzen (1991):

> According to the theory of planned behavior, perceived behavioral control, together with behavioral intention, can be used directly to predict behavioral achievement. At least two rationales can be offered for this hypothesis. First, holding intention constant, the effort expended to bring a course of behavior to a successful conclusion is likely to increase with perceived behavioral control. For instance, even if two individuals have equally strong intentions to learn to ski, and both try to do so, the person who is confident that he can master this activity is more likely to persevere than is the person who doubts his ability. The second reason for expecting a direct link between perceived behavioral control and behavioral achievement is that perceived behavioral control can often be used as a substitute for a measure of actual control. Whether [this can be done] depends, of course, on the accuracy of the perceptions.
>
> (Ajzen 1991: 6)

The first rationale offered by Ajzen refers to a *causal* effect of PBC on behaviour, one that is mediated, not by intention, but by 'effort' and 'perseverance' (neither of which are constructs in the TPB). By contrast, the second rationale refers to what is merely an *association* between PBC and behaviour that is not due to a causal effect of one variable on the other. According to this second rationale – which was the one emphasized by Ajzen and Madden (1986) in an early exposition of the TPB – behaviour is influenced directly by the degree of *actual control* the individual has over the behaviour; perceived control does not influence behaviour directly. If the second rationale is correct and the first is not, it follows that changing PBC in an intervention without changing actual control will not lead to behaviour change directly (though to the extent that PBC influences intention and intention influences behaviour, changing PBC may lead to behaviour change indirectly).

In contrast to the TPB, the TRA is a pure causal model with clearer implications for intervention. Future research on the TPB should measure actual control as well as PBC and should try to estimate the relative size of the causal and non-causal components of the independent predictive effect of PBC on behaviour. This would seem to require laboratory-based experimental studies in which actual and perceived control are manipulated.

A further complication concerns the interactive influence of PBC and intention on behaviour that was postulated by Ajzen and Madden (1986). This interaction derives from an interaction between intention and actual control. In particular, intention is expected to have a stronger influence on behaviour the greater the degree of actual control the person has over the behaviour. Put another way (since interactions are always symmetrical), the effect of actual control on behaviour will be larger the stronger the person's intention to perform the behaviour. Thus, an intervention that increases intention will be more effective in producing behaviour change if actual control is high (or if the intervention also increases the degree of actual control). Similarly, an intervention that increases actual control will be more effective in producing behaviour change if intention is high (or if the intervention also increases intention).

These complexities are peculiar to the TPB. The problems discussed in the remainder of the chapter apply to both the TRA and the TPB. However, because it is the simpler model, the TRA rather than the TPB is used to illustrate the main points.

Although it is not the purpose of this chapter to review intervention studies based on the TRA and the TPB, it is worth noting that surprisingly few studies have followed the sequence of steps outlined above to develop and test a health behaviour intervention. Among the studies that have approximated this sequence are Hoogstraten *et al.* (1985) study on seeking dental treatment, Brubaker and Fowler's (1990) study of testicular self-examination, and Parker *et al.*'s (1996) study on speeding. The reader is referred to Hardeman *et al.* (submitted) for a systematic review of applications of the TPB to behaviour change interventions.

4 Deciding which component to target

The analysis conducted at Step 3 is designed to help the investigator decide which component (attitude or subjective norm) to target in the intervention or whether to target both. The relative size and statistical significance of the regression weights is used to inform this decision. (Alternatively, the unique percentage of variance explained or the squared semi-partial or part correlation may be used; note that the significance test is the same as that for the corresponding regression coefficient.) However, this method assumes, among other things, that attitude does not cause subjective norm and that subjective norm does not cause attitude. But the two components are typically correlated positively with each other, often quite highly. In other words, those people who have a positive attitude towards performing the recommended action also tend to believe that important others would want them to perform it. *This correlation is not explained by the TRA or the TPB.* It could be due to any or all of the following: subjective norm may influence attitude; attitude may influence subjective norm; or another variable or variables may influence both attitude and subjective norm. By estimating the independent predictive effects of attitude and subjective norm on intention (that is, the effect of attitude, controlling for subjective norm, and the effect of subjective norm, controlling for attitude), and interpreting these as causal effects, we are assuming implicitly that attitude does not cause subjective norm and that subjective norm does not cause attitude, in other words that the observed correlation between attitude and subjective norm is due only to the third of the three mechanisms. (This reflects common practice in research on social cognition models: in assessing which of a model's components are the more important determinants of intention or behaviour, researchers usually emphasize the *independent* predictive effects of the components.)

However, the notion that subjective norm influences attitude (or that attitude influences subjective norm) is not implausible. If people believe that significant others want them to perform the behaviour, they may, as a consequence, have a positive attitude towards the behaviour. If so, there will be a positive correlation between attitude and subjective norm, and the beta weight for the independent predictive effect of subjective norm on intention may underestimate the total causal effect. For example, suppose that attitude and subjective norm are correlated 0.50, that the standardized partial regression coefficients (beta weights) are 0.40 for attitude and 0.20 for subjective norm, and that both coefficients are significantly different from zero. This is represented by the first path model in Figure 11.1. The investigator may conclude from this analysis that attitude should be targeted in preference to subjective norm.

But suppose we make the assumption that the correlation between attitude and subjective norm is entirely due to a causal effect of subjective norm on attitude, as represented by the second path model in Figure 11.1. According to this model, subjective norm influences intention both directly and indirectly via attitude. The beta weights for the direct effects of attitude and subjective norm on intention will be the same as in the first model but now the estimated total effect of subjective norm on intention ($= 0.20 + (0.50 \times 0.40) = 0.40$) is equal to the estimated direct effect of attitude. The implication is that it would be a mistake to target attitude and ignore subjective norm. Indeed, changing subjective norm would be one way of changing attitude.

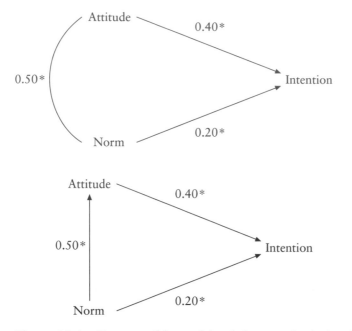

Figure 11.1   Two possible models of the causal relationships between attitude, subjective norm, and intention

Although a number of meta-analyses of the TRA and the TPB have been conducted (for example Sheppard *et al.* 1988; Van den Putte 1993; Godin and Kok 1996; Notani 1998; Armitage and Conner in press), only one, on condom use, reported the correlation between attitude and subjective norm. Albarracín *et al.* (2001) obtained weighted (by sample size) mean correlations of 0.44 between the direct measures of attitude and subjective norm and 0.42 between the indirect measures. It would be helpful if future meta-analyses of the TRA and the TPB followed Albarracín and colleagues by reporting the full matrix of weighted mean correlations.

In drawing implications for intervention from regression analyses of the TRA or TPB, investigators should consider the size and significance of not only the direct effects but also the total effects, under different models of the causal relationship between the predictors. However, given the difficulties involved in deciding which of two correlated components is more important, it can be argued that from a practical viewpoint the best strategy is always to target both. Of course, this strategy becomes less manageable as the number of putative determinants of intention increases, as in extended versions of the Theory of Planned Behaviour (see, for example, Chapters 5, 8 and 9 by Armitage and Conner, Parker, and Evans and Norman in this volume).

5 Selecting the key beliefs

Another problem concerns the selection of key beliefs (Step 4 in the sequence described above). Assume that we have decided to target the attitudinal component. A widely used procedure is to divide the sample in the main study into 'intenders' and 'non-intenders' and to compare these two groups on each of the behavioural beliefs in turn using t-tests. Such analyses may examine belief strength, outcome evaluation, and/or the product term. Those beliefs that best discriminate between the two groups (that is, show the largest, or most statistically significant, difference in means) are selected for the intervention. Alternatively, the sample may be divided on a measure of behaviour or a direct measure of attitude.

This procedure, and the notion that some salient beliefs are more important than others in influencing intention, is actually inconsistent with a key assumption of the TRA and the TPB. Figure 11.2 shows the causal relationships between salient behavioural beliefs, indirect attitude, direct attitude, and intention that are postulated by the TRA and the TPB. For simplicity, we assume that there are only three salient beliefs and that intention is entirely under attitudinal influence, so we can forget about subjective norm and PBC. As Figure 11.2 shows, the models assume that every salient *be* product term has the *same weight* (equal to one) in determining attitude. In other words, all the product terms are *equally important* in determining attitude. Changing any of the product terms by the same amount, while keeping the other terms constant, will produce the same change in attitude, and therefore in intention. Thus, attempting to identify beliefs that are more important than others (for example that show larger differences in means between intenders and non-intenders or larger correlations with intention) is inconsistent with the equal-weighting assumption of the TRA and the TPB.

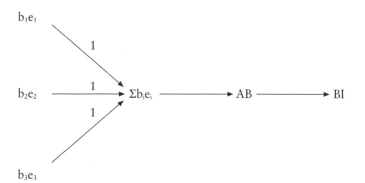

Figure 11.2 Path diagram showing the assumed causal relationships between salient behavioural beliefs (b_1e_1, b_2e_2, b_3e_3), indirect attitude (Σb_ie_i), direct attitude (AB) and intention (BI)

The assumption that the *be* terms for salient behavioural beliefs have equal weights can be tested formally in a hierarchical multiple regression analysis using the simple procedure suggested by Rindskopf (1984). Alternatively, structural equation modelling can be used. In the latter method, a direct measure of attitude or intention would be regressed on the *be* product terms, first allowing the (unstandardized) regression coefficients to be unconstrained and then constraining them to be equal. If the unrestricted model gave an adequate fit (the fit would be perfect if single measures of attitude, or intention, and each of the product terms were used and the latter were allowed to covary freely) and if introducing the equality constraints produced little or no decrement in fit, it would be reasonable provisionally to reject the unrestricted model in favour of the restricted model. In this case, it would be appropriate to consider any or all of the salient beliefs as potential candidates for intervention. If the unrestricted model cannot be rejected, this would provide support for the hypothesis that some beliefs are more influential than others, and those with the larger coefficients could be chosen for intervention. From a theoretical viewpoint, this would constitute evidence against the equal-weighting assumption of the TRA/TPB. It would also raise the question of whether the weights have a psychological interpretation.

Such analyses can become unwieldy if there are too many *be* terms, and problems associated with multicollinearity may arise. Nevertheless, they are more appropriate than the analyses outlined at the beginning of this section which do not test the equal-weighting assumption and do not take the correlations between beliefs into account. A problem that affects both analyses where product terms are used is that the correlations between a multiplicative composite such as *be* and other variables will vary arbitrarily depending on the particular scoring schemes used for its components (Schmidt 1973; Bagozzi 1984; Evans 1991). In principle, it is possible to avoid this problem by combining tests of the equal-weighting and multiplicative assumptions in a hierarchical multiple regression analysis.

Another issue concerns the relationship between modally salient and individually salient beliefs. If a standard set of modal salient beliefs is used, there is no guarantee that these will correspond to the salient beliefs held by a particular individual. Two methods of identifying individually salient beliefs have been used. The first is to ask participants to generate their own beliefs using open-ended questions and then to rate them in terms of belief strength and outcome evaluation (for example Rutter and Bunce 1989; Agnew 1998). The second method is to present participants with a set of modal salient beliefs and ask them to select those that are personally important (for example Van der Pligt *et al.* 2000). Both these methods allow interventions to be individually targeted. Each individual would receive a different version of the intervention, the exact content depending on their own idiosyncratic set of salient beliefs. Although individually tailored interventions have become associated with stage models of behaviour change (for example Prochaska *et al.* 1993), they can also be based on models such as the TRA and the TPB.

6 Effective variance explained

When there are only a few salient beliefs, as in Figure 11.2, changing one of the *be* product terms can make a substantial difference to the indirect attitude score. The more salient beliefs there are, however, a given change in one product term will make a proportionately smaller difference to the attitude score. The implication is that it is likely to be necessary to produce changes in a number of beliefs rather than just one or two.

Even if we succeed in changing indirect attitude or indirect subjective norm, the effect may not carry through to produce a measurable change in behaviour. Meta-analyses show that the TRA and the TPB explain on average 40–50 per cent of the variance in intention and 19–38 per cent of the variance in behaviour (Sutton 1998). In the case of the TRA, the estimates of variance explained in behaviour reflect the effect of intention, the variable that is assumed to be most proximal to behaviour. However, according to the model, it is not possible to intervene directly to change intention. Interventions must be applied to the most distal variables in the model, that is, to beliefs. It is important therefore to estimate the percentage of variance in behaviour explained by the distal variables, which we refer to as the *effective variance explained*. The effective variance explained is rarely reported in studies of the TRA, but it can be easily computed if we know the three correlations between behaviour and the indirect measures of attitude and subjective norm.

Of the meta-analyses referred to earlier, only two reported the effective variance explained or provided information that enables it to be calculated. In the first of these, Van den Putte (1993) estimated that behavioural beliefs (that is, indirect attitude) accounted for only 4 per cent of the variance in behaviour, and normative beliefs (indirect subjective norm) explained only 2 per cent of the variance in behaviour, on average. Van den Putte did not explain precisely how he calculated these estimates but it would seem that he simply multiplied together the weighted mean correlations for each link of the putative causal chain. For example, for the path from indirect subjective norm through to behaviour, the correlations estimated from the meta-analysis were 0.53 for indirect and direct subjective norm, 0.42 for direct subjective norm and intention, and 0.62 for intention and behaviour. This gives a product of 0.138, which is equivalent to 1.9 per cent of variance explained. This is a crude estimate because these correlations were based on different numbers of studies. Furthermore, for various reasons, it is likely to be an *over*estimate of the unique variance explained by indirect subjective norm. In particular, it does not adjust for the effect of indirect attitude (which, as we have already noted, is likely to be positively correlated with indirect subjective norm).

In their recent meta-analysis of 42 studies of the TRA and the TPB applied to condom use, Albarracín and colleagues (2001) reported the full matrix of weighted mean correlations. From these it can be calculated that indirect attitude and indirect subjective norm jointly explain 15 per cent of the variance in condom use and that the unique variance in behaviour explained by each of these components is 5.5 per cent and 3.2 per cent respectively. (Note that, like van den Putte 1993, these authors included studies in their meta-analysis in which behaviour was measured at the same time as attitudes and beliefs.)

For assessing the intervention potential of a model, effective variance explained provides a better basis than the proportion of variance explained by the model as a whole or the proportion explained by the proximal variables. It can also be used to compare the predictive power of different social cognition models. Indeed, when expressed in these terms, the TRA and the TPB may perform little better than the Health Belief Model, which is frequently criticized for its weak predictive power (for example Sheeran and Abraham 1996). Nevertheless, explaining even as little as 5 per cent of the variance in behaviour may represent a useful achievement from a public health standpoint, if the predictor variable in question is modifiable through interventions that have a wide reach and if we can be reasonably confident that the observed association is due to a causal effect of the predictor on behaviour (Sutton 1998).

Also useful for gauging the intervention potential of social cognition models are measures of effect size based on the partial regression coefficients. In their meta-analysis, Albarracín et al. (2001) reported path analyses based on the matrix of weighted mean correlations. The effects of indirect attitude and indirect subjective norm on behaviour (condom use) can be calculated from the path coefficients reported in their Figure 11.2. For example, in their analysis of TRA studies, the effect of indirect attitude on behaviour, controlling for indirect subjective norm, was 0.16. In other words, assuming that the causal sequence postulated by the TRA is correct, if indirect subjective norm is held constant, an increase of one standard deviation unit in indirect attitude would be expected to produce an increase of 0.16 standard deviation units in behaviour. The corresponding effect of indirect subjective norm on behaviour, controlling for indirect attitude, was 0.04. These effects can be compared with the path coefficient of 0.57 for the effect of intention on behaviour, controlling for the antecedent variables in the model.

Although it is conventional in this field to report standardized coefficients, the unstandardized coefficients may be easier to interpret for some purposes. The unstandardized effect of indirect attitude on behaviour gives the expected change in behaviour when indirect attitude is increased by one unit, where both variables are measured in their original units and indirect subjective norm is held constant. (The interpretation of unstandardized coefficients is particularly simple when the behaviour measure is a 0–1 dichotomy. Suppose the unstandardized coefficient for the effect of indirect attitude is 0.20. This means that the probability of performing the behaviour is expected to increase by 0.20 when indirect attitude is increased by one original unit and indirect subjective norm is held constant.)

It should be noted that the problem we mentioned earlier concerning multiplicative composites also applies to the preceding discussion.

The implication of the causal dilution that occurs as we move from the distal variables through to behaviour is that, even if an intervention is successful in producing a change in indirect attitude or subjective norm, the effect on behaviour may be very small (although, as we have pointed out, even small effects may be useful from a public health viewpoint). This in turn implies that large samples may be required to detect the effects of an intervention. Researchers who plan to develop and test health behaviour interventions based on the TRA or the TPB should always conduct analyses of statistical power and precision to estimate the required sample size.

7 Changing beliefs

Assuming that the other problems we have discussed can be overcome, the TRA and the TPB can be used to identify a small number of beliefs to be targeted in an intervention. But they do not specify how to change such beliefs. Fishbein and Ajzen have supplemented their expositions of the TRA with detailed discussions of the cognitive processes involved in persuasion and have made a useful distinction between descriptive, informational and inferential beliefs (for example Fishbein and Ajzen 1975; Fishbein *et al.* 1980; Fishbein and Ajzen 1981). However, as Eagly and Chaiken (1993: 240) note, even with these extensions 'the model provides no formal guidance for choosing arguments to include in messages designed to influence a specific belief'. This is an important limitation of the TRA and the Theory of Planned Behaviour, which they share with most other social cognition models used in the health behaviour field. A possible exception is social cognitive theory/ self-efficacy theory (Bandura 1997) which specifies ways in which the key variable of self-efficacy can be enhanced, for example through guided mastery experiences.[2]

The currently dominant dual-process theories of persuasion also offer little help in this regard. According to the Elaboration Likelihood Model (Petty and Cacioppo 1986; Petty and Wegener 1999), the kind of change in beliefs or attitudes that is usually regarded as desirable in the health behaviour field (that is, enduring, resistant to counterpersuasion and predictive of behaviour) is most likely to be produced if a communication presents strong arguments and if the recipients are able and motivated to think about and elaborate on these arguments. However, little research has been done on what constitutes a 'strong' argument; empirical studies using the ELM rely heavily on pretesting to identify high quality arguments. Furthermore, relatively few studies have used the theory in the context of health behaviour change; the typical ELM study investigates attitudes to issues or policies such as a proposed increase in tuition fees rather than beliefs or attitudes with respect to changing personal health behaviour.

8 Conclusion

This chapter has identified a number of problems in using the TRA and the TPB to develop health behaviour interventions. The discussion highlights the need for more basic research on the assumptions underlying the models and on the processes that mediate belief change. Key questions that need to be addressed include:

1 What is the relative size of the causal and non-causal components of the independent predictive effect of PBC on behaviour?
2 What are the mechanisms that produce the correlations between the theoretical determinants of intention?
3 In the light of these processes, what is the relative size of the causal effects of these factors on intention?
4 What is the most appropriate way of defining and measuring salience, and how can salient beliefs best be identified?
5 Do the equal-weighting and multiplicative assumptions adequately describe the way that salient beliefs are combined?
6 What are the mechanisms underlying belief change?
7 What makes an argument 'strong' rather than 'weak'?
8 Is it possible to integrate theories of persuasion with theories of attitude-behaviour relations?

Until progress is made in resolving these issues, the potential of the TRA and the TPB as tools for developing effective behaviour change interventions is likely to remain largely unfulfilled.

Notes

1 In theory, behaviour change can also be produced or facilitated by modifying the strength of the causal links in the TRA. However, with the possible exception of the intention-behaviour link, little work has been done using this approach, so this chapter will focus on changing beliefs as the principal intervention strategy.

2 Given the similarity between the self-efficacy and PBC constructs, it can be argued that the same methods could be used to change PBC. From the standpoint of the TPB, any change in PBC must be mediated by changes in salient control beliefs. It would be interesting to use the TPB measures to assess the effects of guided mastery experiences.

References

Agnew, C.R. (1998) Modal versus individually-derived beliefs about condom use: measuring the cognitive underpinnings of the theory of reasoned action, *Psychology and Health*, 13: 271–87.

Ajzen, I. (1991) The Theory of Planned Behavior, *Organizational Behavior and Human Decision Processes*, 50: 179–211.

Ajzen, I. and Fishbein, M. (eds) (1980) *Understanding Attitudes and Predicting Social Behavior*. Englewood Cliffs, NJ: Prentice-Hall.

Ajzen, I. and Madden, T.J. (1986) Prediction of goal-directed behavior: attitudes, intention, and perceived behavioral control, *Journal of Experimental Social Psychology*, 22: 453–74.

Albarracín, D., Johnson, B.T., Fishbein, M. and Muellerleile, P.A. (2001) Theories of reasoned action and planned behavior as models of condom use: a meta-analysis, *Psychological Bulletin*, 127: 142–61.

Armitage, C.J. and Conner, M. (in press) Efficacy of the theory of planned behaviour: a meta-analytic review, *British Journal of Social Psychology*.

Bagozzi, R.P. (1984) Expectancy-value attitude models: an analysis of critical measurement issues, *International Journal of Research in Marketing*, 1: 295–310.

Bandura, A. (1997) *Self-Efficacy: The Exercise of Control*. New York: Freeman.

Brubaker, R.G. and Fowler, C. (1990) Encouraging college males to perform testicular self-examination: evaluation of a persuasive message based on the revised theory of reasoned action, *Journal of Applied Social Psychology*, 17: 1411–22.

Conner, M. and Norman, P. (eds) (1996) *Predicting Health Behaviour: Research and Practice with Social Cognition Models*. Buckingham: Open University Press.

Eagly, A.H. and Chaiken, S. (1993) *The Psychology of Attitudes*. New York: Harcourt Brace and Jovanovich.

Evans, M.G. (1991) The problem of analyzing multiplicative composites: interactions revisited, *American Psychologist*, 46(1): 6–15.

Fishbein, M. and Ajzen, I. (1975) *Belief, Attitude, Intention and Behavior: An Introduction to Theory and Research*. Reading, MA: Addison-Wesley.

Fishbein, M. and Ajzen, I. (1981) Acceptance, yielding and impact: cognitive processes in persuasion, in R.E. Petty, T.M. Ostrom and T.C. Brock (eds) *Cognitive Responses in Persuasion*. Hillsdale, NJ: Erlbaum.

Fishbein, M. and Middlestadt, S.E. (1989) Using the theory of reasoned action as a framework for understanding and changing AIDS-related behaviors, in V.M. Mays, G.W. Albee and S.F. Schneider (eds) *Primary Prevention of AIDS: Psychological Approaches*. Newbury Park, CA: Sage.

Fishbein, M., Ajzen, I. and McArdle, J. (1980) Changing the behavior of alcoholics: effects of persuasive communication, in I. Ajzen and M. Fishbein (eds) *Understanding Attitudes and Predicting Social Behavior*. Englewood Cliffs, NJ: Prentice-Hall.

Godin, G. and Kok, G. (1996) The Theory of Planned Behavior: a review of its applications to health-related behaviors, *American Journal of Health Promotion*, 11(2): 87–98.

Hardeman, W., Johnston, M., Johnston, D. *et al.* (submitted) Application of the theory of planned behaviour in behaviour change interventions: a systematic review.

Hoogstraten, J., De Haan, W. and Ter Horst, G. (1985) Stimulating the demand for dental care: an application of Ajzen and Fishbein's theory of reasoned action, *European Journal of Social Psychology*, 15: 401–14.

Notani, A.S. (1998) Moderators of perceived behavioral control's predictiveness in the theory of planned behavior: a meta-analysis, *Journal of Consumer Psychology*, 7: 247–71.

Parker, D., Stradling, S.G. and Manstead, A.S.R. (1996) Modifying beliefs and attitudes to exceeding the speed limit: an intervention study based on the theory of planned behavior, *Journal of Applied Social Psychology*, 26(1): 1–19.

Petty, R.E. and Cacioppo, J.T. (1986) The elaboration likelihood model of persuasion, in L. Berkowitz (ed.) *Advances in Experimental Psychology*, 19. London: Academic Press.

Petty, R.E. and Wegener, D.T. (1999) The elaboration likelihood model: current status and controversies, in S. Chaiken and Y. Trope (eds) *Dual-process Theories in Social Psychology*. New York: Guilford.

Prochaska, J.O., DiClemente, C.C., Velicer, W.F. and Rossi, J.S. (1993) Standardized, individualized, interactive, and personalized self-help programs for smoking cessation, *Health Psychology*, 12(5): 399–405.

Rindskopf, D. (1984) Linear equality restrictions in regression and loglinear models, *Psychological Bulletin*, 96: 597–603.

Rutter, D.R. and Bunce, D.J. (1989) The theory of reasoned action of Fishbein and Ajzen: a test of Towriss's amended procedure for measuring beliefs, *British Journal of Social Psychology*, 28: 39–46.

Schmidt, F.L. (1973) Implications of a measurement problem for expectancy theory research, *Organizational Behavior and Human Performance*, 10: 243–51.

Sheeran, P. and Abraham, C. (1996) The health belief model, in M. Conner and P. Norman (eds) *Predicting Health Behaviour*. Buckingham: Open University Press.

Sheppard, B.H., Hartwick, J. and Warshaw, P.R. (1988) The Theory of Reasoned Action: a meta-analysis of past research with recommendations for modifications and future research, *Journal of Consumer Research*, 15: 325–39.

Sutton, S. (1998) Predicting and explaining intentions and behavior: how well are we doing?, *Journal of Applied Social Psychology*, 28(15): 1317–38.

Van den Putte, B. (1993) On the theory of reasoned action. Unpublished doctoral dissertation, University of Amsterdam.

Van der Pligt, J., de Vries, N.K., Manstead, A.S.R. and van Harreveld, F. (2000) The importance of being selective: weighing the role of attribute importance in attitudinal judgment, in M.P. Zanna (ed.) *Advances in Experimental Social Psychology*, 32. New York: Academic Press.

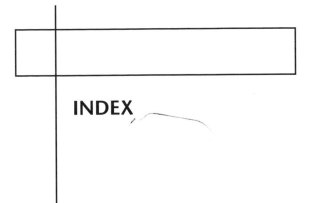

INDEX

CONTROL AND THE PSYCHOLOGY OF HEALTH
THEORY, MEASUREMENT AND APPLICATIONS

Jan Walker

- What is meant by 'control' in the psychology of health?
- How do different control-related concepts relate to each other?
- How can control be measured?

This ambitious and much needed text presents a comprehensive review of theories and concepts that are central to our understanding of the psychology of health, including perceived control, locus of control, learned helplessness, self-efficacy and social support. The origin and theoretical development of each concept are explored, and the links between them analysed. Their current status as variables in health-related research is examined and examples of their applications in a variety of health care contexts are given, along with an overview of tools of measurement. The final chapters bring these concepts together within a single theoretical framework, which explains the potential interaction of personal control and social support in promoting and sustaining psychological well-being. For student courses, this book will enhance the understanding of control theory and its relevance to health behaviour change and health care interventions. In addition, it will aid conceptual clarity and measurement for those wishing to design research based on the concept of control.

Contents
Summary of control concepts – Perceived or personal control – Locus of control – Self-efficacy – Learned helplessness – Social support – Emotional states – A unifying theory of control – References – Index.

272pp   0 335 20264 0 (Paperback)   0 335 20265 9 (Hardback)

Learning
(

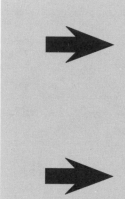